I have only known Dr. Janet Maccaro for two years, but I can say that I am most impressed with all she is doing to help hurting people feel better. I had the opportunity to work with her on a health telethon in Los Angeles, and I immediately saw the tremendous potential she had as a "media doctor."

We plan to host a weekly television with her that will air on our Hollywood Television Network—a national television and cable network geared to the senior's marketplace. We anticipate great results from this new show with Janet as host.

Congratulations, Janet, on your new book, *90-Day Immune System Makeover.* I wish you much success in this exciting project. I am sure it will meet many needs.

—PAUL S. WEBB, CHAIRMAN AND CEO
HOLLYWOOD TELEVISION NETWORK

How to live longer, better and forever—this has been the goal for our *Today's Family* program for over eighteen years. Health and nutrition information is so important for every member of the family. Dr. Janet Maccaro brings a refreshing yet simple message that we can be all God wants us to be by looking after our "temples" before health problems are diagnosed.

Janet has been a regular guest on our programs and has helped many of our viewers and TV-52 staff members. Her approach makes nutrition and health easy to understand. She helps us to see that God has made us, and by applying His principles, we can live life more abundantly.

I know this book will be a big help to those who, like me, are looking for answers to make lifestyle and nutritional changes. A must-read for anyone who is serious about their health!

—KEN MIKESELL, PRESIDENT AND GENERAL MANAGER
WTGL-TV 52
ORLANDO, FLORIDA

D1016071

I feel honored to have been asked to participate in this manner in Janet's book. She has been, and is, very special to me. She gives of herself so freely, and I am one of the recipients of that giving nature. It seemed to me that my physical being, and consequently my life, was out of control with hormone imbalances and hypoglycemia. The symptoms I experienced were hot flashes, mood swings and frequent and drastic blood sugar drops, which resulted in anxiety and what I call the "foggy brain syndrome." My day-to-day living experience was quite an effort. Through Janet's guidance, I started using Stevia for my hypoglycemia and progesterone cream for my hot flashes. Along with proper diet, a cleansing routine at least twice a year and nutritional support to keep my immune system at optimum, most days are wonderful for me—unless I ruin it with my choice of food. I am very grateful.

All of Dr. Janet Maccaro's life experiences, including debilitating illnesses and extreme hormone inbalances, have influenced her path into nutritional counseling. She gives of herself above and beyond the call of duty because she cares. Today there are tremendous health challenges for many. Dr. Maccaro guides and educates those who seek her counsel in an understanding of how improved nutrition, the use of food supplements and natural hormone balancing can improve the quality of their lives.

She is a very special friend to me and brings spirituality, caring and compassion to all with whom she comes in contact. Thank you, Janet.

—SARA WEINER, OWNER
LIVING WATERS HEALTH FOODS

90-DAY
IMMUNE
SYSTEM
MAKEOVER

90-DAY
IMMUNE
SYSTEM
MAKEOVER

Janet C. Maccaro, Ph.D., C.N.C.

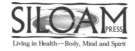

SILOAM PRESS

Living in Health--Body, Mind and Spirit

90-Day Immune System Makeover by Janet Maccaro, Ph.D.
Published by Siloam Press
A part of Strang Communications Company
600 Rinehart Road
Lake Mary, Florida 32746
www.creationhouse.com

Unless otherwise noted, all Scripture quotations are from the King James Version of the Bible.

Scripture quotations marked AMP are from the Amplified Bible. Old Testament copyright © 1965, 1987 by the Zondervan Corporation. The Amplified New Testament copyright © 1954, 1958, 1987 by the Lockman Foundation. Used by permission.

Scripture quotations marked NIV are from the Holy Bible, New International Version. Copyright © 1973, 1978, 1984, International Bible Society. Used by permission.

Scripture quotations marked NKJV are from the New King James Version of the Bible. Copyright © 1979, 1980, 1982 by Thomas Nelson, Inc., publishers. Used by permission.

Scripture quotations marked RSV are from the Revised Standard Version of the Bible. Copyright © 1946, 1952, 1971 by the Division of Christian Education of the National Council of the Churches of Christ in the USA. Used by permission.

Library of Congress Catalog Card Number: 00-102254
International Standard Book Number: 0-88419-692-5

This book is not intended to provide medical advice or to take the place of medical advice and treatment from your personal physician. Readers are advised to consult their own doctors or other qualified health professionals regarding the treatment of their medical problems. Neither the publisher nor the author takes any responsibility for any possible consequences from any treatment, action or application of medicine, supplement, herb or preparation to any person reading or following the information in this book. If readers are taking prescription medications, they should consult with their physicians and not take themselves off of medicines to start supplementation without the proper supervision of a physician.

0 1 2 3 4 5 6 7 VERSA 8 7 6 5 4 3 2 1
Printed in the United States of America

In my quest for wellness many people were placed in my path. Some were an inspiration, others teachers, and last, but not least, some have become dear friends who have witnessed the transformation in my life and how God is truly faithful!

First on my list is my husband, Michael, who has stood by me as a sounding board, supporter and encourager through twenty-three years of marriage. To my children, Michael, Amanda and Jillian, who may have not understood me very well during my years of health challenges. I love you!

To Dr. Karen Hayter for her friendship and listening heart.

To Charlie Fox of Wakunaga for believing in my mission and connecting me to wonderful opportunities.

To Ken Mikesell and his staff at WTGL-TV 52 in Orlando, Florida, for giving me the opportunity to share from the heart time and time again on *Today's Family*. I thank you for launching my career.

To David Self of Cosmed Labs for helping to develop and launch Dr. Janet's Balanced by Nature products.

To Sara Weiner of Living Waters Health Foods for all of her support and friendship over the past few years. Love you, Sara.

To MEDIA Power, especially John Buckley for all of the radio bookings, even at 6 A.M., and Chris, Carol and Ken for giving me an opportunity to work in the MEDIA.

To all of my clients.

To Bethel Ministries and John Jeyaseelan and his wife, Hema, for their continual prayerful support.

To my best friend, Barbara Wolfe-Lee, for all of the laughter we've shared throughout the years. Laughter is truly one of the best medicines. Our friendship is God's gift to us!

To Paul Webb, chairman and CEO of the Hollywood Television Network, for being a support, sounding board and friend.

To all of my clients, it has truly been a blessing to work with each of you. It gives me great joy to see each one of you achieve a higher level of health. Now you can go forth and teach others what you have applied.

Finally, to Siloam Press and Rick Nash and staff for this opportunity to get my message of health, hope and healing out to the multitudes of men and women who are struggling as I once did.

DISCLAIMER

90-Day Immune System Makeover has been written and published strictly for informational purposes. In no way should it be used in place of the advice of your own health care provider.

You should not consider the educational material in the Makeover to be the practice of medicine, although much research has been done and clinical experience has shown positive results time and time again. In addition, the information from patient trials, anecdotes, testimonials and patient histories is from health care professionals and has been utilized to educate and empower the reader with the knowledge of natural methods to boost immunity and to prevent needless suffering. This book provides you with the latest and time-tested natural alternatives to strengthen your body, mind and spirit. Because this book is for educational purposes only, Dr. Maccaro recommends an ongoing dialogue with your health care professional.

CONTENTS

Contents

LIST OF CHARTS

AUTHOR'S NOTE

This book is a culmination of the last thirty years of my life—years filled with many health challenges and pain. I often wondered and cried out to God, *Why me?* Did I do something, or did I hurt someone? Even New Agers tried to tell me it was some karmic debt I had to pay in this lifetime.

Enter Jesus Christ. My whole world changed, answers came and prayers were answered. Not only was I helped, but many others were also helped by what I learned. It is now crystal clear to me that the Lord *allowed* me to experience all of the following: Epstein-Barr virus, chronic fatigue syndrome, systemic candida yeast infection, hormonal imbalance, eczema, panic attacks, severe strep infections and endometriosis. Now at this appointed time when these diseases are epidemic in proportion, God is using me to help men and women overcome disease as I did and become the true expression of what He intends them to be. For this, I am grateful.

Beloved, I pray that you may prosper in all things and be in health, just as your soul prospers.

—3 John 2, NKJV

SANCTIFY, O LORD,

those whom You have called

to the study and practice of the

Arts of Healing and to the prevention

of disease and pain. Strengthen them by

Your life-giving spirit that by their

ministries the health of the community

may be promoted and Your creation

glorified, through Jesus Christ our Lord.

—AUTHOR UNKNOWN

FOREWORD

Wow! The human race has turned over another millennium! Congratulations to us! We are progressing in almost every area of our lives, and we seem to believe that things are just going to get better and better. We believe our economy is sound, we are focusing in on family, and we say we are taking better care of ourselves. We pride ourselves on our health care facilities, our exercise commitments and our low-fat diets. Americans are obsessed with health and living healthy, and we appear to believe that "when you have your health, you have everything." And yet, we remain one of the sickest nations in the world, in almost every sense of the word.

Why are we so sick? Perhaps because we have long been a nation that treats the symptoms, not the cause. We would rather pop a pill than work on the underlying problems. We want to be healthy, but we also want a quick fix and really don't want to have to work for it.

Welcome to the *90-Day Immune System Makeover*, a concept whose time has come and that will give us health naturally and quickly. More and more people are discovering the benefit of getting healthy in a natural manner, as evidenced by the popularity of health food stores, nutritionists, whole-food grocery stores and magazines about health. It seems that in addition to an accountant, a lawyer, a doctor and a therapist, everyone wants to have a nutritionist these days. The *90-Ninety Day Immune System Makeover* will give you that nutritionist, Dr. Janet Maccaro, and will also provide you with her expertise on making your immune system effective and efficient in keeping you healthy.

Someone has suggested that a weakened immune system is the doorway to all disease. Therefore, it is of vital importance to strengthen and fortify your immune system. When you have a strong immune system, and you choose to take supplements, you will reap the greatest benefit from them. And if some nasty bug or virus tries to take you out of commission, you will have the best "lean, mean, fighting machine" available to do combat for your body. That's what an immune system working at peak performance can do.

So, where do you start? Congratulations! You have already started by reading this book. Dr. Maccaro will tell you about her own difficult struggle to achieve good health. She will describe for you how to get your body cleansed of harmful elements, how to get your hormones in balance and the best way to get your lymphatic system and adrenal glands working. She will teach you how to cleanse your body of harmful elements, what to eat, when to eat, what supplements are best for you and how to stay healthy all of your life. Her passion for helping people be healthy and live up to their potential in all areas of life is evident in her life and on these pages. Follow this program, and you will achieve additional health, better relationships, feel better about life in general and feel better about yourself—as well as have more energy to do the things you have always wanted to do. What could be better than that?

Ninety days will pass by anyway, whether you do something about your health or not. Why not make the commitment to yourself today to do something really good for you? Get that immune system in shape and get healthy!

—Dr. Karen Johnson Hayter
Producer/Host
COPE

INTRODUCTION

In the new millennium, our immune systems will be under constant attack from newer and more powerful bacterial and viral microbes. I believe that the frequent use of antibiotics combined with increased levels of pollution, stress and poor eating habits have left us in a state that I call a low level or sub-level of health. I believe many people are functioning at this sub-health level while trying to survive mentally, physically, financially and, most importantly, spiritually. Living in a state of sub-health means that your immune system is weakened, which translates into increased susceptibility to disease.

In this book, I will share with you my 90-Day Immune System Makeover. I have used it to regain my health after chronic fatigue syndrome, as have hundreds of my clients when faced with body imbalance. I consider it the best weapon against immune dysfunction. God has provided us with powerful compounds from nature that have the ability to boost immune function so we can effectively battle viral, parasitic and bacterial invaders. We can be mentally, physically and spiritually "armed and dangerous" against the attacks on our physical bodies in this new millennium. If you would like to safeguard your health and rev up your immune system, read on, and I will teach you about building your immunity and avoiding the immune system zappers that we face. After reading *90-Day Immune System Makeover,* you will be well equipped with the knowledge to protect yourself against them.

> My people are destroyed for lack of knowledge.
> —Hosea 4:6

Here we are in the year 2000.

We see that we are living in times unlike any other. For example:

- More children under the age of fifteen are lost through the terminal process of cancer than by any other cause, with the exception of accidents.
- Degenerative diseases are not limited to senior citizens. All ages are now affected.
- According to the Senate Nutrition Committee, cardiovascular diseases are the leading cause of death in the United States. One out of every two Americans suffer from heart disease.
- According to the American Heart Association, thirty-seven million people suffer from high blood pressure.
- According to the Nutrition Research Alternatives Report, over eleven million people in our country suffer from diabetes.

2

- One-third of the American population is overweight, so much so that their life expectancy is reduced. This is because they are more prone to high blood pressure, high cholesterol and high blood sugar levels, which in turn lead to heart disease, diabetes and hypertension.
- Tooth decay affects over 90 percent of the population under the age of seventeen. Forty-five percent of the population suffer from periodontal disease, the leading cause of tooth loss over the age of fifteen.
- Since 1967, roughly seven billion dollars have been spent on cancer research. In 1950, the cancer rate was one out of fifteen. Today the figure is one out of four. This represents 25 percent of our population.
- In 1950, mental illness affected one out of twenty people. It is now said that one in five will be affected.

This 90-day program teaches you to remove all obstacles to true health and balance, thereby allowing your God-given potential for healing to manifest. During the first 30 days, you will detoxify your body and eliminate sugar, caffeine, wheat, dairy and alcohol. You will learn about the importance of water. You will eat healthier for energy and blood sugar balance. This first phase of the 90-Day Immune System Makeover is a cleansing, re-balancing and preparation phase. You will be laying the foundation for a super strong immune system. We will begin with your immune health screening to identify your weaknesses, whether hereditary or self-imposed.

The 90-Day Immune System Makeover has both short-term and long-term effects and will serve as your road map to optimal immunity and a higher quality of life. The short-term benefit is that you will feel better as you implement the principles of the program. The long-term effect is that you will achieve maximum immunity in order to avoid or battle a chronic or even potentially life-threatening disease in the future. This journey I have walked before you. I have been the patient before I became the doctor. I can tell you that regaining my health was the most incredible journey that I have ever experienced. I pray that as you embark on this program you also experience healing in your body, mind and spirit.

God, in your wonderfully designed body, made your immune system as the greatest pharmacy in the world. Your immune system makes more than one hundred billion types of medicines, called antibodies, to attack just about any unwanted germ or virus that enters your body. It is what keeps you healthy and makes you well after a viral, bacterial or fungal infection. It can even manage to stop a cancer cell from setting up shop in your body and multiplying.

Most importantly, all the medicines made by your internal pharmacy are completely natural and custom tailored to work specifically for you. They do not produce side effects, they are free, and they are the most powerful healing agents known to man.

Your immune system has one requirement—the right raw materials to produce the internal medicines needed for you to remain healthy.

This will be the only technical portion of the *90-Day Immune System Makeover*. I call this section Basic

Introduction

Immunity 101. Think of your immune system as your own personal army, always on guard and ready to defend your body twenty-four hours a day, seven days a week for the entire course of your life. Now more than ever we require a vigilant and vigorous immune system with the many new and more powerful microbes and pathogens in our environments.

Your immune system is designed to recognize a substance as "self" or "non-self" or a potential enemy. If a substance is recognized as an invader, like in the case of a bacteria, yeast or fungi, unrecognized by the body's own code, the immune system's army must take swift action and make war against it. An important part of your immune system's troops called *macrophages* come in to engulf or eat foreign cells or molecules. Macrophage, which is derived from a Greek term meaning "big eater," can be likened to Pac-Man eating and attacking invaders. Macrophages use weapons known as free radicals and enzymes that virtually weaken the intruder. Once weakened and dissolved, the macrophages completely digest the invader, thereby stopping the invasion from becoming more deeply entrenched in the body. This is known as a "nonspecific defense mechanism" because every invader is treated equally by macrophages.

However, if macrophages find that the battle is too much for them to handle, then more specialized troops must be called in for battle. This is where T cells come in to take further action and render the intruder harmless. The T cells, also known as T suppressors, are responsible for halting the immune system's attack when the battle is over. Other divisions in your immune army include bone marrow, the spleen and lymph nodes. In addition, you have B cells that produce antibodies to attack invaders or antigens, thereby weakening them and leaving them for the macrophages to come in and digest the unwelcome guests.

One of the most incredible things about your immune system's army is that deeply embedded in its memory is the victory against an invader, like chickenpox, measles, mumps and others, which in turn boosts or prolongs your resistance against another attack from the same invaders. As you read each section of the *90-Day Immune System Makeover* you will see the same theme throughout. To keep your immune army in tiptop shape, it's imperative to eat right, sleep enough, exercise daily and supplement your diet with substances that will enhance immune function.

YOUR IMMUNE SYSTEM

T cells are produced by the thymus gland. They destroy virus and cancer cells.	The skin is one of your immune system's first line of defenses.
Macrophages are found in lymph nodes, where they filter foreign particles.	Lymph nodes act as filters.
	The thymus gland produces T cells and releases hormones.
The liver produces lymph and contains Kupffer cells that filter yeasts, toxins and bacteria.	The spleen destroys cellular debris, worn-out blood cells and bacteria. It also acts as a blood reservoir.
B cells produce antibodies that damage invaders or alert white cells to attack.	Bone marrow produces white cells that attack yeasts, viruses, parasites and fungi.

YOUR IMMUNE SYSTEM ARMY AT A GLANCE

GOOD FORCES	ENEMY FORCES
Antibodies–immune proteins that attack invaders	Antigens–invaders
Antioxidants–help the body stop the harmful free radicals	Free radicals–by-products that harm cells
Interferon–protein that helps cells resist infection	Infection–inflammation caused by invaders
T cell–organizes immune response	Pathogen–disease-causing microbe
Macrophage–engulfs invaders	
Lymphocyte–disease-fighting white blood cell made by lymph nodes	
Leukocytes–fight infection	
T helpers–cells that support immune response	
White blood cells–fight infection	
Natural killer cell–a T cell that is especially powerful in eliminating cancerous cells	

By learning about your immune system and how it works, you will be armed with the knowledge you need to stimulate and support its functions, especially during times of stress, poor eating, lack of sleep and negative thinking. You will learn techniques on how to fortify yourself in times of stress, you will learn how to detoxify to lighten the load on your immune system, and you will learn what nutrients will support your wonderful immune system. Also, the renewing of your mind is imperative if you are to reverse negative thoughts that can suppress immunity.

ARE AMERICANS HEALTHY?

By definition, health is "freedom from disease." This implies that if you aren't suffering from a disease, you are healthy.

Americans accept this definition of health. We generally believe that people are healthy if they are free from disease. The aches and pains, stomach problems, insomnia, anxiety, depression and other little annoyances are so common in this country that we accept them as natural occurrences that can be attributed to the aging process. Not so! This 90-Day Immune System Makeover will show you that a strong vibrant body with a robust immune system is possible. It will give you a blueprint or a step-by-step program for reversing those feelings of weakness and diminished vigor so common to Americans today. Optimum immune health will aid in restoring joy in your life.

Good nutrition is the key. By this I mean right foods, whole foods, herbs, vitamins, minerals, amino acids and detoxification. Using ingredients God has provided since the "original garden" can pave the way for vibrant health, eliminating the obstacles to true immune health. To be free of disease, strong in living and joyful in feeling truly well sounds wonderfully familiar, doesn't it?

> Beloved, I pray that you may prosper in all things
> and be in health, just as your soul prospers.
> —3 JOHN 2, NKJV

We are living in the days spoken of when "knowledge shall be increased." Every day publications spout a new wonder drug or "magic bullet" to heal our bodies and cure our anxious minds. Herbs, enzymes, vitamins, lotions, potions and more all claim to be the only way to health. Every day I receive phone calls from or see clients who have been searching for the answer to their physical woes. We have entered a generation of chronic illness. I believe this is due to many factors, namely stress and poor diets laden with junk food, fast food, sodas, dyes, preservatives, hormones and artificial sweeteners. These substances do not build healthy cells, and they are not what God intended for us to ingest, especially not on a daily basis! Now, many have entered health food stores seeking help after the medical profession has failed them.

The medical profession has made tremendous strides in the past forty years, and I am not faulting modern medicine. I have seen many modern miracles that medicine has achieved. But as I mentioned earlier, we are a generation of the chronically ill. Too many people are treated for symptoms of chronic illness continually with medications that have side effects. These medications disrupt the delicate natural balance that God has created in our bodies.

LIFE REPLENISHES LIFE

All life depends upon food; humans are no exception. We must learn to make discriminating choices between what we must and must not eat. The people of this world who have little food must choose carefully in order to survive. Though Americans have an abundance, we must also choose our foods carefully because so much of it is of little or no nutritional value. Ironically, the percentage of people in America suffering from malnutrition is incredibly high.

The abundance of choice in our supermarkets has contributed to our ills. We need to choose live foods that rot or sprout. Most Americans do not shop along the perimeter of the supermarket where live foods are located. People are drawn to the fast preparation foods, loaded with chemicals, preservatives, food colors, artificial flavors and dyes. Most of these foods are dead, lifeless foods. Life replenishes life. God gave us live foods, and they are essential to live in health. Recently while shopping, I spotted a packaged food product with so many chemicals and artificial ingredients that the shelf life printed on the package read 2005! I don't know about you, but I will not put something into my body that will not break down for at least five years! What will those preservatives do to our internal organs? The choices you make every week in the grocery store can make the difference between vibrant health and energy or disease and a shortened life span. You actually make a choice between health and disease each week as you push your cart down the supermarket aisle. To summarize, if it doesn't rot or sprout...do without!

MY STORY

I am very happy that you have made the decision to follow my 90-Day Immune System Makeover program. This program was born out of my own struggle with immune dysfunction. It is the blueprint I used to regain my health. I pray that it is a real blessing to you and that it helps you to build your immune health to the highest level possible. I'd like to begin by sharing my story with you. When I work with clients, I feel it is important for them to know me and how I work.

I was born in Syracuse, New York, and grew up in Florida. For as long as I can remember, bouts of tonsillitis and strep were my constant health challenge four times a year. My doctor prescribed countless antibiotic medications for me (remember, I grew up in the "antibiotic era"). When I was ten, he even prescribed preventive antibiotic treatments to be taken every day indefinitely to help prevent rheumatic fever! As time went on, my father and mother divorced, and my immune system took a nose dive. I was only thirteen, and emotionally and physically, I suffered. I developed shingles, eczema, bowel problems and nervous tics. Not a pretty picture. Still I strove to be the best student, the best friend, the best everything—which only put more stress on me and my immune system.

In my teen years, I modeled, loved fashion design and had dreams of acting and a television career. But my health always got in the way. At eighteen, I had an emergency tonsillectomy, lost twenty-seven pounds and had a systemic yeast infection. I decided then that a job in the health profession was more practical so I could learn more about health. That's when I became a dental assistant. It was fun and rewarding, but I never felt well. I thought it would pass eventually. However, I was never completely well.

Let's fast forward to age twenty when I married my husband, Michael. He was a new dentist, and I was his assistant, hired to help build his new practice. From the first day I met Michael, I knew he would be my husband. Three weeks after working together, it was clear that we were meant to be together. Michael proposed, and six months later we were husband and wife. But still, I did not feel well.

Three months after marriage, we were excited to find out that I was pregnant. Surprisingly, I felt absolutely wonderful, but that came to a crashing halt after I gave birth by C-section to my first child, Michael Joseph. Shortly after I stopped breastfeeding him, I fell into a deep, dark postpartum depression that lasted almost eighteen months. It was as if my life were over at age twenty-one. Finally, after months of searching, we found an endocrinologist in Augusta, Georgia, who diagnosed my problem—severe hormonal imbalance likely brought on by stress. I began hormone shots to gain the proper balance. But my workaholic, A-type personality maintained my stress and made balance almost impossible. In spite of how awful I felt, I continued caring for my family, always doing, going and praying for help.

After my second child, Amanda, was born, yeast infections and additional hormonal problems made life almost unbearable. I started my own quest for health because I knew I had to be well for my children. I often felt sorry for Michael. He married a young, vibrant twenty-year-old, and before his eyes, I became this person who never felt good. I realize how helpless he must have felt during these first years because nobody knew what to do for me.

I continued to have mysterious symptoms that baffled the best doctors. I could recall how wonderful I felt during pregnancy and how awful I felt afterward. Yet I couldn't stay pregnant for the rest of my life! I thought there had to be a reason that pregnancy seemed to restore me to my old self, but the answer eluded me.

Three years later my last child, Jillian, was born by C-section. Her lungs were full of fluid. I hemorrhaged and could not see her for forty-eight hours. I learned that Jillian had the same condition that John F. Kennedy's infant son, Patrick, had died from. When I prayed beside Jillian's neonatal crib in the hospital, I asked God to spare her and promised that I would dedicate the rest of my life to serving Him in a mighty way. God heard my prayer. Jillian survived, and I brought her home.

However, my joy was overshadowed by the same physical ailments. At one point, I had over twenty symptoms. To help keep my mind off of my physical complaints, I became an aerobics instructor and took Jillian with me, and at night, I would entertain at retirement homes with a group of women. One morning, I had to teach a 9 A.M. aerobics class, and when I tried to get out of bed, I couldn't. My body would not let me. I was scared, and I panicked. I cried, *Why, Lord? How much more can I take?* Day after day, I struggled to function. I was totally exhausted, worn out and just plain pooped! Whatever this was, it had a tight grip on me. It was devastating. I had to crawl to change Jillian's diaper. It was a struggle to do anything, especially with three children to care for.

I was disillusioned with the medical profession by this time, but I had to find out what was wrong. The diagnosis came back as Epstein-Barr virus, commonly known as chronic fatigue syndrome. My doctor had no answer; he just monitored me. This was not acceptable. There had to be an answer—a solution. I prayed and prayed and prayed some more. Suddenly I was deluged with people, books, television shows, products, radio shows and magazine and newspaper articles relating to my condition.

I began using natural alternatives to build my immune system, and my strength gradually returned. I used detoxification, herbs, massage, juicing and, of course, prayer. I also learned that progesterone was responsible for the feeling of well-being during my pregnancy and that by supplementing my body afterward created a perfect balance! It took one year to rebuild my system,

14

and during that year all of the questions I had were answered, especially the *Why me?* question. I then went back to school at age thirty-eight and received a Ph.D. in nutrition and a degree in natural medicine so that I could get the message of hope, healing and body balance out to God's people in a mighty way!

Regaining my health was not easy. It took prayer, discipline, determination and focus. The goal of this book is to teach you how to strengthen your immune system in 90 days. Why 90 days? The answer is simple. It takes this long to implement changes and go through detoxification and gain body balance. Just 90 days. This is a short time when you consider the many years of poor living and bad dietary habits you have to undo. God made our bodies incredibly forgiving. If we remove all of the obstacles to true healing from our systems, our bodies will do what they were designed to do...HEAL! So many diseases are carved with our own knife and fork. With proper lifestyle changes, diseases can go right back where they came from. Praise God!

PART ONE:

The First 30 Days

THE FIRST
30 DAYS

In my journey toward wellness, detoxification played a large part in my recovery. No matter what health condition you are facing, even if you feel you are in great health, detoxification is essential to take you to a higher level of health. When I felt my body grow stronger just from cleaning up my diet, I felt I was ready for detoxification.

DETOXIFICATION

When I was very ill, it was hard to detoxify my body because my organs of elimination were not up to par. I had to be very gentle with my system. I learned this the hard way. I consumed cleansing herbs and teas that were simply too much for my weakened system. I suffered severe detox symptoms—vomiting, severe headaches and back and kidney pain—and extreme fatigue, which required bed rest.

If you are dealing with a systemic illness, as I did, your

body first requires pure, whole foods, as close to the original garden as possible. If it did not rot or sprout, I did without. I eliminated dairy and wheat from my diet, as these were too much for my weak body and digestive system. I drank plenty of fresh spring water with fresh lemon every day. Most importantly, I eliminated sugar. It has been said that refined sugar paralyzes the immune system. I was a sugar-holic, and it zapped my body!

According to Leon Chaitow, N.D., D.O., of London, England:

> A body with a healthy immune system, efficient organs of elimination and detoxification, and a sound circulatory and nervous system can handle a great deal of toxicity. But if they have been damaged from chronic exposure to environmental pollutants, restoring these functions, organs, and systems can be accomplished only through detoxification therapies, including fasting, chelation, and nutritional, herbal, and homeopathic methods, which accelerate the body's own natural cleansing processes. These therapies will dominate medical thinking in the years ahead.

Most Americans feel they are simply too busy to take the time to detoxify. People take better care of their cars than they do their physical bodies, and I find this upsetting. Detoxification is a way to clean our bodies and rid them of toxins and debris accumulated over the years. This gives us a clean slate from which to build upon. Just like caring for our car engine, filter, hoses, and so on, our bodies and our "filter"—the liver—need cleansing. How do you know if you need to detoxify?

The following indicators are common in people who are in need of detoxification.

- Poor elimination
- Junk food
- Overeating or stress eating
- Fatigue
- Aches and pains
- Rashes
- Insomnia
- Bad breath

- Poor diet
- Sugar
- Lack of water
- Stress
- Use of antibiotics
- Lack of exercise
- Late night eating

How did you do? If you can relate to any of these symptoms, detoxification will be a blessing to you and will give you the best start to a stronger immune response.

Initially, I used colonics (a series of six). This is up to you. I believe they are beneficial but not essential. Colonics, or colon therapy, is an effective way to cleanse the large intestine of toxins and waste products. It functions to draw toxins out of the blood and lymph and back into the colon for excretion. A colonic is simply having a hose inserted rectally that has warm water running through it. This "washes" the inside of your entire intestinal tract.

You can find colonic therapists in your area, most often by asking an alternative health doctor for a recommendation. Colonics can be used prior to other detoxification programs.

If you choose to start with a series of colonics, be sure to supplement your intestinal tract with a bowel flora formula such as acidophilus or bifidus. Colonics can strip healthy bowel flora while cleansing away toxins and encrusted matter in the intestines. You may purchase bowel flora formulas at health food stores.

If colonics do not appeal to you, try Lindsey Duncan's Nature's Secret Ultimate Cleanse. (There are other cleansing systems on the market, but I have found this to be the best.) This formula has been a real blessing to myself, my family and the hundreds of people I have worked with over the past several years. I wish I had access to this product years ago when I struggled with poor bowel function and digestive difficulties because of the ease, gentleness and effectiveness of the product. This is a two-part program that cleanses all of your channels of elimination.

If you choose to use Nature's Secret, it will take you about thirty days to complete the two bottles that are in the box. At the same time, drink plenty of non-chlorinated water and eat a diet that is as close to the original garden as possible: no preservatives, refined sugars, cakes, pies, cookies, candy, soda, caffeine, dairy, alcohol or wheat. This product offers immediate results by gently supporting the body's natural eliminative processes of two to three bowel movements per day. I recommend that you detoxify two times a year—once in the spring and once in the fall.

If you have never implemented a detoxification program before, be advised that as your body begins to "clean house" you could develop headaches, flu-like symptoms, aches and pains, nausea and skin eruptions. These are all positive signs that it's working. All of the past is being discarded. After a few days or weeks on a detoxifying program, your mind will be clearer, your energy will soar, you will have better digestion, your skin will glow, and you will sleep better. In essence, you will feel like a new person. After a good detoxification program, you really are a new person!

TIPS DURING DETOXIFICATION

- Take an acidophilus supplement daily. I recommend Kyo-Dophilus by Wakunaga.
- Buy a loofah or natural bristle skin brush and brush your skin (away from the heart) before showering each day. This will assist the elimination process through the skin.
- Drink plenty of quality water—six to eight glasses daily.
- Engage in mild exercise such as walking, stretching or bike riding.
- Take a salt and soda bath. A list of therapeutic baths for specific conditions is given in the next section.

Skin brushing can be very beneficial because the skin is a primary avenue for detoxification, along with the lungs, kidneys, liver and colon. Use a vegetable brush, purchased from a health food store. Brush all parts of the body away from the heart. Then follow with a sesame oil massage. Massaging with sesame oil brings relief. This oil can also be purchased from a health food store. Massage the whole body for five minutes before bathing or showering.

Baths for purification

You may experience flu-like symptoms during the detoxification because your body is ridding itself of poisons. You can get relief from these symptoms by taking baths using sea salts (1 to 2 cups) and baking soda (1 cup) in a tub of water and soaking for twenty minutes (more than twenty minutes may exhaust you). This bath also counteracts the effects of radiation, whether from x-rays, cancer treatment radiation, fall-out from the atmosphere or television radiation. On off days, you can put one cup of apple cider vinegar in the tub and soak. Here are some other baths you can use:

- Clorox bath: This will help to remove heavy metals from the body and add oxygen. Use ½ cup Clorox brand bleach, use ONLY this brand, to a tub of warm water. Soak for twenty-five minutes. You can shower off with soap and fresh water afterward, but it is not necessary. If your skin feels a bit itchy, this will relieve it.

- Epsom salts and ginger: This bath opens pores and eliminates toxins and relieves pain. Stir in 1 cup Epsom salts and 2 tablespoons of ginger to a cup of water first, then add it to the bath. Do not remain in the tub for more than thirty minutes.

- Epsom-sea-oil: This bath helps with dry skin and stress. Put 1 cup Epsom salts, 1 cup sea salt (from health food store) and 1 cup sesame oil into a warm to hot tub of water, and then soak for twenty minutes. Pat yourself dry.

- Vinegar bath: This is used when the body is too acidic and is a quick way of restoring the acid-alkaline balance. Mix 1 cup to 2 quarts of 100 percent apple cider vinegar to a bathtub of warm water. Soak forty to forty-five minutes.

This is excellent for excess uric acid in the body and for the joints, arthritis, bursitis, tendonitis and gout.

· Bentonite bath: This is a fast detoxification method. Soak 2 to 4 pounds of bentonite clay in a flat container overnight to dissolve it. Then add the dissolved clay to a tub of water. With 2 pounds of bentonite, soak one hour; with 4 pounds, soak only about thirty minutes. The more bentonite used, the faster the detoxification.

IMMUNE RESPONSE

As we embark upon the first 30 days of the 90-Day Immune System Makeover, it is imperative that you take inventory of your body and see just where your weaknesses are. You may find that some of your complaints seem to run in your family or are hereditary. Don't let this alarm you. Remember, "to be forewarned is to be forearmed." This simply means that those weak areas need more attention or strengthening. It is essential to discover and live principles of healthful living that will restore balance to the immune system.

While overcoming my personal health struggles, my studies took me on a journey through all avenues of alternative medicine. In Chinese medicine, it is believed that if you have moved into chronic illness of any kind, a balancing principle must be applied. That is, all five systems of our bodies—respiratory, endocrine, digestive, circulatory and immune—must be balanced. This balancing is known as the principle of regeneration. Regeneration differs from medicine because it has nothing at all to do with disease. To treat a disease, medicine first names it, then seeks a specific cure for it. The regeneration principle, in contrast, holds that there are no specific diseases, only internal weaknesses, usually reversible, that manifest in certain symptom patterns. By using the symptom pattern to discern the weakness, then strengthening the body system, we create optimal conditions that allow the symptoms to go away, replaced by the vitality and balance of health. The regeneration principle was a blessing to my physical body.

> My people are destroyed for lack of knowledge.
> —HOSEA 4:6

On the following page you will find your immune response questionnaire. This is your immune system barometer to let you know where your strengths and weaknesses lie. We will repeat this questionnaire at the end of the makeover. As you circle your current symptoms, keep firmly in mind that you must shift your thinking from the disease-oriented point of view, seeking an external cure for a specific disease, to a regeneration principle point of view, seeking to strengthen and balance your body and paying attention to symptoms only as signs of possible weakness. Vitamins, medicines, herbs, potions and lotions heal nothing! God made our bodies with the ability to heal. The 90-Day Immune System Makeover will support the body, strengthen the weak areas and let the healing begin!

IMMUNE RESPONSE QUESTIONNAIRE

Instructions: Please circle the number that best describes the frequency or severity of your complaints. Leave the question blank if it does not apply to you.

0 = no symptoms	2 = moderate symptoms
1 = mild symptoms	3 = severe symptoms

Section A

1. Easily susceptible to infections	0	1	2	3
2. Frequently catch a cold or flu	0	1	2	3
3. Difficult to recuperate from a flu or cold	0	1	2	3
4. Chronic swollen lymph glands	0	1	2	3
5. Frequent sore throats	0	1	2	3
6. Cuts or bruises heal slowly	0	1	2	3
7. Hair grows slowly	0	1	2	3
8. Frequent ear infections	0	1	2	3
9. Cold sores or fever blisters	0	1	2	3
10. Chronic low-grade fever	0	1	2	3
11. Gums and/or nose bleeds easily	0	1	2	3
12. Experience frequent runny nose	0	1	2	3
13. Muscle aches and joint pain	0	1	2	3

Section B

1. Known chemical sensitivities	0	1	2	3
2. Known environmental and/or food allergies	0	1	2	3
3. Irritability/mood swings	0	1	2	3
4. Frequent headaches and/or migraines	0	1	2	3
5. Abnormal fatigue not helped by rest	0	1	2	3
6. Postnasal drip	0	1	2	3
7. Frequent sneezing attacks and/or hayfever	0	1	2	3
8. Weight fluctuations of four to five pounds in one day accompanied by puffiness in face/ankles/fingers	0	1	2	3
9. Chronic muscle aches and pains	0	1	2	3
10. Suffer from asthma/breathing difficulties	0	1	2	3
11. Eczema, hives or skin rashes	0	1	2	3
12. Suffer from depression or crying spells	0	1	2	3
13. Itchy eyes or nose	0	1	2	3
14. Chronic runny nose	0	1	2	3

15. Chronic stuffy nose	0	1	2	3
16. Dark circles under your eyes	0	1	2	3
17. Frequent urination or bedwetting	0	1	2	3
18. Swelling in joints	0	1	2	3
19. Mouth or throat itches	0	1	2	3
20. Chronic lymph gland swelling, especially in the throat area	0	1	2	3
21. Acne	0	1	2	3
22. Sweat for no apparent reason/hot flashes	0	1	2	3
23. Suffer from irritable bowel, spastic colon or colitis	0	1	2	3
24. Certain foods cause you to have a reaction (jitters, depression, ill feeling)	0	1	2	3
25. Strong cravings for certain foods	0	1	2	3
26. Pulse races after eating certain foods or for no apparent reason	0	1	2	3
27. Mucus in stool	0	1	2	3
28. Minor, chronic complaints that always reoccur	0	1	2	3
29. Feel best when you do not eat	0	1	2	3
30. Hyperactive	0	1	2	3
31. Abdominal pain after eating	0	1	2	3
32. Alternating diarrhea/constipation	0	1	2	3

Section C

1. Chronic fatigue, especially after eating	0	1	2	3
2. Depression	0	1	2	3
3. Recurrent digestive complaints	0	1	2	3
4. Rectal itching	0	1	2	3
5. Food and/or environmental allergies	0	1	2	3
6. Severe PMS	0	1	2	3
7. Feel "spacey"	0	1	2	3
8. Poor memory	0	1	2	3
9. Severe mood swings	0	1	2	3
10. Anxiety/nervousness	0	1	2	3
11. Recurrent fungal infections (athletes foot, ringworm, jock itch)	0	1	2	3
12. Extreme chemical sensitivity	0	1	2	3
13. Cannot tolerate perfumes or smoke	0	1	2	3
14. Coated or sore tongue	0	1	2	3

15. Prostatitis	0	1	2	3
16. Recurrent vaginal or urinary infections	0	1	2	3
17. Lightheadedness or feeling drunk after minimal wine, beer or certain foods	0	1	2	3
18. Respiratory problems	0	1	2	3
19. Chronic skin rashes or acne	0	1	2	3
20. Loss of libido/impotence	0	1	2	3
21. Thrush	0	1	2	3
22. Headaches/migraines	0	1	2	3
23. Muscle and joint pains	0	1	2	3
24. Low blood sugar	0	1	2	3
25. History of frequent antibiotic use	0	1	2	3
26. Taking or have taken birth control pills	0	1	2	3
27. Crave sugar, breads or alcoholic beverages	0	1	2	3
28. Endometriosis and/or infertility	0	1	2	3
29. Above conditions get worse in moldy places like basements or damp climates	0	1	2	3
30. Above conditions get worse after eating or drinking items that contain yeast or sugar	0	1	2	3

Section D

1. Fatigue	0	1	2	3
2. Depression	0	1	2	3
3. Anxiety	0	1	2	3
4. High blood pressure	0	1	2	3
5. Increased susceptibility to infections	0	1	2	3
6. Headaches	0	1	2	3
7. Digestive problems (colic, nausea, pain)	0	1	2	3
8. Numbness/tingling/tremors	0	1	2	3
9. Skin problems (rashes, eczema, psoriasis)	0	1	2	3
10. Learning disabilities	0	1	2	3
11. Ringing in your ears	0	1	2	3
12. Muscle and joint pain	0	1	2	3
13. Allergies/asthma	0	1	2	3
14. Kidney and/or liver problems	0	1	2	3
15. Constipation	0	1	2	3
16. Memory problems	0	1	2	3
17. Anemia	0	1	2	3
18. Varied symptoms with no relief	0	1	2	3

In the quest for my own physical regeneration, I discovered a fascinating chart developed by Dean Black, Ph.D., author of *Health at the Crossroads,* based on the regeneration principle. Over the years, I have adapted it to common vitamins, minerals and herbs. As you read the list of health challenges, keep in mind that you are not treating or curing your ailment, but rather strengthening the systems of your body that most likely are responsible for your condition. I have listed each health condition and beside it have numbers with the corresponding system most responsible for the condition according to the regeneration principle. You may want to explore the possibility of strengthening your weakened areas, detoxifying your body and following the immune-eating plan to have regeneration take place in your own body. Suggested supplements can be found in the Body-Strengthening Chart, which follows the Health Challenges Chart. It was a wonderful experience for me. Remember, your health challenge did not occur overnight, so it will take time for the process of regeneration to take place. Most of my clients notice a difference in 90 days. This is why I have included it in the *90-Day Immune System Makeover.* These guidelines show you what areas that need to be strengthened by proper supplementation, diet, exercise and, of course, prayer.

HEALTH CHALLENGES CHART

KEY: Number 1 is the system mostly weakened and involved in disease. Number 2 is the next weakened area that is involved in disease. Number 3 is the third system that is involved. Number 4 is the fourth.

ACNE	ADDICTION
1 Endocrine System 2 Circulatory System 3 Immune System 4 Digestive System (start with detox and immune-eating plan)	1 Nervous System (start with detox and immune-eating plan)

ALLERGIES	ARTHRITIS (RHEUMATOID)
1 Endocrine System 2 Respiratory System 3 Immune System 4 Digestive System 5 Circulatory System (start with detox and immune-eating plan)	1 Endocrine System 2 Immune System 3 Circulatory System 4 Nervous System (start with detox and immune-eating plan)

ASTHMA	AUTO-IMMUNE CONDITIONS
1 Respiratory System 2 Endocrine System 3 Circulatory System (start with detox and immune-eating plan)	1 Endocrine System 2 Immune System 3 Circulatory System (start with detox and immune-eating plan)

BLADDER INFECTIONS	BLOOD PRESSURE
1 Endocrine System 2 Immune System (Cranberry capsules/daily drink plenty of water/eliminate sugar)	1 Circulatory System 2 Endocrine System 3 Fat Regulation

BOWEL PROBLEMS	CANDIDA ALBICANS (YEAST)
1 Digestive System 2 Circulatory System (start with detox and immune-eating plan)	1 Immune System 2 Female Hormone 3 Endocrine System 4 Digestive System (start with detox and anti-yeast diet with antifungal)

CHOLESTEROL	COLD
1 Digestive System 2 Circulatory System 3 Fat Regulation	1 Respiratory System

31

COLITIS	CONGESTION
1 Digestive System (start with detox immune-eating plan)	1 Respiratory System 2 Endocrine System 3 Immune System 4 Digestive System 5 Circulatory System

DEPRESSION	DIABETES
1 Endocrine System 2 Female Hormone 3 Nervous System (detox, exercise, immune-eating plan) Please consult your physician if your condition is more than mild!	1 Circulatory System 2 Endocrine System

DIGESTIVE DISTURBANCES	ECZEMA
1 Digestive System	1 Endocrine System 2 Immune System (start with detox and immune-eating plan)

EMOTIONAL INSTABILITY	ENDOMETRIOSIS
1 Nervous System 2 Endocrine System 3 Female Hormone (for women)	1 Endocrine System 2 Female Hormone 3 Immune System 4 Respiratory System

FATIGUE	FEVER
1 Nervous System 2 Fat Regulation (start with detox, immune-eating plan)	1 Immune System 2 Respiratory System (Liquid diet—fruit juices, broths to give your system a break from digestion so fever clears faster)

GOUT	HEADACHE
1 Immune System 2 Circulatory System 3 Endocrine System (detox, eliminate animal protein, immune-eating plan)	1 Nervous System 2 Respiratory System 3 Circulatory System (detox, immune-eating plan)

HEARTBURN	INDIGESTION
1 Digestive System (detox, immune-eating plan)	1 Digestive System (detox, immune-eating plan, take digestive enzymes with meals)

INSOMNIA	LUPUS
1 Nervous System 2 Digestive System 3 Circulatory System (start with detox and immune-eating plan)	1 Endocrine System 2 Respiratory System 3 Immune System 4 Digestive System (Begin with immune-eating plan; when strong enough, a gentle detox will cleanse the body of toxins, making you feel much better.)
MENSTRUAL CRAMPS	**MENOPAUSE (HOT FLASHES)**
1 Female Hormone 2 Endocrine System (calcium, magnesium, natural progesterone cream)	1 Female Hormone 2 Endocrine System
MIGRAINE HEADACHES	**NERVOUS WEAKNESS**
1 Nervous System 2 Endocrine System 3 Respiratory System 4 Circulatory System (detox, immune-eating plan, magnesium)	1 Nervous System 2 Circulatory System 3 Endocrine System (detox, immune-eating plan, calcium, and magnesium)
SINUS	**SORE THROAT**
1 Respiratory System 2 Endocrine System 3 Immune System (detox, immune-eating plan, eliminate dairy and wheat)	1 Respiratory System 2 Immune System (detox, immune-eating plan, zinc lozenges)
STRESS	**WEIGHT CONTROL**
1 Nervous System 2 Endocrine System	1 Fat Regulation (detox, immune-eating plan: weight loss is a natural result)
WRINKLES	
1 Endocrine System 2 Female Hormone (limit exposure to the sun)	

BODY-STRENGTHENING CHART

The following supplements are support for strengthening the body systems below:

DIGESTIVE	CIRCULATORY
Digestive enzymes	Omega 3 Oils
Liquid chlorophyll or Kyo-Green	Coenzyme Q_{10}
Acidophilus	Ginger
Dandelion	Cayenne
Ginger	Garlic
Chamomile	Bilberry
	Ginko biloba

NERVOUS SYSTEM	FAT REGULATION
B-complex with extra pantothenic acid	B-complex
Passionflower	Carnitine
Kava	Chromium picolinate
Valerian	Exercise
Calcium	Liver glandular
Magnesium	
Royal jelly	
Amino acids	

RESPIRATORY	IMMUNE
Fenugreek	IP6
Reishi mushroom	Reishi mushroom
Beta carotene	Kyo-Green
Garlic	Astragalus
Cayenne	Vitamin A
Selenium	Vitamin C
Ginger	Vitamin E
Vitamin A	Echinacea
Vitamin C	Garlic
Vitamin E	Acidophilus
Zinc	Maitake
Beta glucans	Siberian ginseng
	Royal jelly

ENDOCRINE	FEMALE HORMONE
Adrenal gland supplement	B-complex
B-complex	Black cohosh
Green drink	Natural progesterone cream
Calcium	Dong quai
Magnesium	Vitex
Chromium picolinate	

WATER

Many people in this country suffer from aches and pains, constipation, skin eruptions and fatigue. You may find it hard to believe, but a lack of water is often behind some of these common complaints. Our society consumes coffee by the gallons and soft drinks and iced tea by the liters. "Plain old water" for some people is just plain boring. Many clients inform me on their first visit that they don't drink water, but they make sure they drink enough liquids each day. I ask them to tell me what liquids they drink. You guessed it. Iced tea, coffee, concentrated juices and soft drinks! I often see clients who ingest large quantities of vitamin supplements every day with a glass of iced tea or soda! No wonder these people are having problems!

Water makes up 65 to 75 percent of our bodies. It is second only to oxygen for our survival. Water helps to flush wastes and toxins, regulates body temperature and acts as a shock absorber for joints, bones and muscles. It cleanses the body inside and out. It transports nutrients, proteins, vitamins, minerals and sugars for assimilation. When you drink enough water, your body works at its peak. Many of my clients who have a problem with water retention, edema and bloating are simply not drinking enough water. Once they do, these symptoms improve. If you are trying to lose weight, you should know that when you drink enough water, hunger is curtailed. To maintain the proper function of your system, you must start drinking good, clean water every day.

The recommended amount is six to eight glasses per day. If this seems like a lot to you, just start slow. Add a slice of fresh lemon, and you will get even more of a cleansing benefit. In addition, it's easier to drink more with a hint of flavor from a lemon. This always works for my clients who used to believe that they could never increase their water intake. Now, I see these people out and about with a bottle of water in their hand. This only proves that they now know how much better they feel just by drinking enough water. They are now so convinced that they carry it with them.

Once people catch the importance of drinking water, the next question is, What *kind* of water is best for drinking? This is a good question since most of our tap water is chlorinated, fluoridated or treated to the point of being an irritant to the system instead of a blessing. Many toxic chemicals have found their way into ground water, adding more pollutants to our water supply. This growing concern about water purity has led to the huge bottled water industry. Many stores today have whole aisles dedicated to bottled water.

Let's go over the different types of water to clear up any confusion. First, we have mineral water, which most often comes from a natural spring with naturally occurring minerals and a taste that varies from one spring to the next. Naturally occurring minerals found in mineral water help to aid digestion and bowel function. Europeans have long known the benefits of bottled mineral water. California and Florida regulate the purity of mineral water produced in their states.

Next, we have distilled water. You may have known someone who believes that drinking distilled water is the only way to go. I disagree. While it is true that distilled water is probably the purest water available, it is de-mineralized. I believe that drinking de-mineralized water on a long-term basis is not ideal. I believe that you need the minerals that naturally occur in water. While distilled water is a good cleanser and detoxifier, I don't believe it is a good builder because it is devoid of minerals. If you are on a detoxifying program or on chemotherapy, distilled water is excellent to remove debris and toxins. After you are finished with detox or chemotherapy, then return to drinking a good mineral or spring water to insure proper mineral activity.

Sparkling water is another choice that comes from natural carbonation in underground springs. Most of them are artificially boosted in carbonation by carbon dioxide to maintain a longer fizz. Many people enjoy sparkling water after dinner to aid in digestion.

Today water filters are available that attach to your kitchen sink faucet to remove impurities as they flow out of the tap. You may also have seen water pitchers with filters that purify the water as you fill the pitcher. I feel these two inventions are quite necessary to help improve the quality of the water we consume. I feel both options are acceptable for building health. Whatever type of water you choose, the most important thing to remember is that you must pay conscious attention to getting your quota of water every day. Thirst is not a reliable signal that your body needs water. You can easily lose a quart or more of water during activity before you even feel thirsty. Also, remember that caffeine and alcohol are diuretics. They increase your body's need for water. If you consume caffeine or alcohol, please make sure you drink enough water to compensate. Ideally, caffeine and alcohol do not belong in a health-building program.

In addition to making sure that your water intake is optimal, take the time to quench your spiritual thirst.

> Whosoever drinketh of the water that I shall give him shall never thirst; but the water that I shall give him shall be in him a well of water springing up into everlasting life.
>
> —JOHN 4:14

WATER WISDOM

To help educate you on water filtration, here is a chart that will make you an authority on the subject.

FILTER TYPE: DISTILLATION

Cost: $800–4,500 for whole house system
$600–1,100 for free-standing unit
$100–$1,000 for countertop model

How they work: Boils water, leaving contaminant behind. This purified water vapor is then condensed to a liquid.

What they reduce: Chromium, lead, nitrates, sulfate, giardia, arsenic, cadmium

FILTER TYPE: REVERSE OSMOSIS (KNOWN AS "RO" WATER)

Cost: $600–1,500 for under-the-sink model
$150–200 for countertop model

How they work: Pressurized water is forced through a purifying membrane that eliminates contaminants; purified water then goes to a holding tank.

What they reduce: Radium, chromium, iron, cadmium, color, chlorine, lead, radium, giardia, sulfate

FILTER TYPE: CARBON FILTRATION

Cost: $25–30 for faucet model
$350–up for under-the-sink model

How they work: Water is passed through a carbon or charcoal block, which traps contaminants. Filters must be replaced periodically.

What they reduce: Chlorine, odors, chemicals, pesticides, bad taste

FILTER TYPE: WATER SOFTENER

Cost: $1,000–3,500

How they work: Sodium (rock salt) is used to soften the water.

What they reduce: Calcium, radium, iron

SUGAR

Sugar consumption inhibits immune function, starting just thirty minutes after consumption and lasting for more than five hours. One hundred grams of sugar in any form—honey, table sugar, fructose or glucose—can reduce the ability of your immune system's army to engulf and destroy invaders. Instead of consuming sugar for energy as so many Americans do daily, consume complex carbohydrates like whole-grain bread, rice or potatoes. These foods will not suppress your immune system but will boost your energy. Sugar is also a food we reach for in times of stress or tension. This is especially detrimental to our health because it makes our system acidic and strips our stabilizing B vitamins. As lifestyles become more and more hectic, people consume more and more sugar. Excessive sugar consumption has been shown to suppress the immune response, lowering our resistance to disease.

There are other ways to add sweetness to your life. I use stevia extract instead of white table sugar. You may also use the following sweet substances in moderation: honey, date sugar, maple syrup and fructose. For something really sweet that really satisfies, get into the Word of God. This is especially true if you feel that you have a sugar addiction. Sugar gives you a lift that eventually brings you down lower than where you started. The Word of God will never let you down.

Diseases that are known to be caused in part by excessive sugar consumption are hypoglycemia and diabetes. Hypoglycemia is extremely common these days. I feel this is due to the high-carbohydrate, high-sugar foods that we crave in our stressful lives; in addition, we consume little or no fiber. This type of eating overloads the pancreas. In turn, insulin is overproduced to lower the blood sugar, which translates into low blood sugar or hypoglycemia. If you are consuming too much sugar on a daily basis, you may set yourself up for hypoglycemia. Here is a list of the common symptoms associated with low blood sugar:

- Rapid pulse
- Crying spells
- Heart palpitations
- Anxiety
- Twitching
- Exhaustion
- Weakness
- Cold sweats
- Irritability
- Poor concentration
- Fatigue
- Nightmares

If these symptoms are familiar to you, you must eat more fiber and protein foods at each meal, and cut back on simple sugar. It is imperative that you have a protein snack between meals. This will keep your blood sugar levels stable all day long.

Diabetes occurs when all of the sugar and carbohydrates that a person consumes are not used properly. The pancreas no longer produces insulin, creating high blood sugar. This can be very dangerous. According to the U.S. Department of Health and Human Services, more than twenty million people suffer from diabetes in this country. Diabetes can lead to heart and kidney disease, stroke, blindness, hypertension and even death. Jonathan Wright, M.D., recommends that diabetics totally eliminate refined sugar and sugar products from their diet.

Eliminating sugar during these first 30 days will not

be easy. Sugar is very addictive. Here are some dietary addition suggestions to make the adjustment easier.

- Chromium picolinate
- B-complex
- Vitamin C
- Protein shake each morning
- High fiber—for example, brown rice
- Stevia extract as an herbal sweetener
- Pantothenic acid
- Adrenal gland supplement
- Calcium and magnesium

Since low blood sugar can predispose you to developing diabetes later in life, take this short quiz to see if your sugar consumption may not only be affecting your level of health now, but later on as well.

1. Do you have a family history of diabetes?
   ❑ Yes   ❑ No
2. Do you crave sweets at certain times of the day?
   ❑ Yes   ❑ No
3. When you are under stress, do you crave sweets?
   ❑ Yes   ❑ No
4. Do you consume ice cream, chocolate, pies, cakes and candy more than twice a week?
   ❑ Yes   ❑ No
5. Do you feel weak and shaky if your meal is delayed?
   ❑ Yes   ❑ No
6. Do you feel tense, uptight and nervous at certain times during the day?
   ❑ Yes   ❑ No
7. Do you crave sodas or other sweetened soft drinks?
   ❑ Yes   ❑ No
8. Do you pay attention to low-fat foods while ignoring the higher sugar content typically found in them?
   ❑ Yes   ❑ No

If you answered yes to four or more of these questions, your excess sugar consumption may be sending you into low blood sugar, or hypoglycemia. This condition is responsible for many uncomfortable symptoms that can ruin the quality of your life. In addition, you may become diabetic later on from a pancreas that is simply too worn out to produce the necessary insulin that is crucial for controlling blood sugar levels.

Sugar has also been implicated in the leading cause of death in America, heart disease. People who consume a high-sugar diet can develop high levels of blood fats, triglycerides and cholesterol. I have found out that in my clients with high triglycerides, sugar was their daily treat. Once these clients were educated on the dangerous risk of heart disease from having a sweet tooth, they cleaned up their diets faster than you can imagine. Also, fat does not make you fat. Sugar does. Yes, sugar is stressing your entire body daily, making you feel tired and irritable, and most importantly contributing to a future of chronic disease.

No sugar? But how?

Your first 30-day eating plan has blood sugar balance in mind. In addition to the eating plan, I always include chromium picolinate, 200 micrograms if you weigh up to 150 pounds. If you weigh more than 150 pounds, add another 200 micrograms, for a total of 400 micrograms in divided doses. Chromium will help you as you wean yourself off of these addictive substances that have been robbing you of your health. You'll be interested to know that people who consume these dietary no-no's and who are under constant stress are typically low in chromium.

Oftentimes I have seen my clients experience a heightened sense of well-being after eating the 30-day eating plan and taking chromium picolinate. I have also found that chromium seems to increase energy levels. I believe this is because of the blood sugar balancing effect on the body. The energy peaks and valleys disappear and are replaced with an even, sustained energy. In addition to chromium, I recommend pantothenic acid, which is a B vitamin that helps the body handle stress. This vitamin does wonders for your adrenal glands that are so often zapped by caffeine, sugar, lack of sleep and stress.

Pantothenic acid and chromium picolinate will help you make the lifestyle changes you need to experience a healthier immune system. And instead of sugar, I recommend stevia extract to sweeten teas or anything that requires sweetening. You will find it to be a wonderful blessing that is noncaloric and is safe for diabetics and hypoglycemics.

Why eliminate artificial sweeteners?
America has jumped on the artificial sweetener bandwagon because of our obsession and preoccupation with weight. It seems like a simple answer for those trying to watch their sugar calories. But simple it is not! One of the components of aspartame is methanol, considered toxic even in small amounts. Toxic levels of methanol have been associated with brain swelling and inflammation of the heart muscle and the pancreas—even blindness! I recommend that you read *Aspartame: Is It Safe?* by H. J. Roberts. In it you will read about reports of convulsions, memory loss, mood swings, headaches, nausea and more. It is also implicated in fetal brain damage. Therefore,

pregnant and lactating women and very young or allergy-prone children should avoid aspartame. By the way, methanol is also known as wood alcohol. Why would you even consider putting this into your body?

Remember that we are trying to eat as close to the original garden as possible. This means natural or close to its original form. Aspartame is made synthetically. There are natural whole-food sweeteners that can satisfy your occasional sweet tooth without risk to your health. The natural sweeteners permitted on the immune system makeover program are:

- Honey—twice as sweet as sugar. Avoid honey if you are diabetic or have candida or low blood sugar. It contains vitamins and enzymes.
- Rice syrup—40 percent as sweet as sugar and is made from rice and water.
- Sucarat—a natural sweetener made from sugar cane juice. It is a concentrated sweetener that should be used with caution if you have blood sugar imbalance.
- Stevia—an herb from South America that can be used in beverages, baking and cooking. Safe for persons with blood sugar imbalances and/or candida and diabetes. Stevia is available as a liquid extract or white powered extract. This happens to be my favorite.
- Fructose—twice as sweet as sugar, derived from fruit. Do not use fructose if you have candida.

DAIRY PRODUCTS

Cow's milk is for baby calves. The only milk we should

consume is our own mother's milk when we are infants. It has been proven that mother's milk helps to fortify an infant's immune system during the first year of life. Did you ever notice that baby calves drink their mother's milk only for a short period of time to get the wonderful benefits? After a certain age, they stop nursing and receive all the calcium and minerals they need by eating the green grass in the cow pasture.

I simply do not recommend drinking cow's milk or using cow's milk in cooking when I have a client on a healing program. Cow's milk has clogging and mucus-forming properties. This is counterproductive when you are trying to cleanse your system. Dairy foods can also interfere with the detoxification process because of the high-fat content. I believe that we can receive calcium that is better absorbed by our bodies from vegetables, sea vegetables, nuts, seeds and fish.

Since dairy foods are obstacles that prevent optimal immune function, they must be eliminated. Dairy products interfere with the initial cleansing and healing process because they are dense, system-clogging, mucus-producing and hard to digest for a large segment of the population. Nondairy alternatives will provide you with the positive aspects of dairy with none of the negative.

During these first 30 days, you will eliminate dairy products and replace them with healthy nondairy alternatives. Many adults and children today are lactose-intolerant and cannot easily digest cow's milk. In addition, cow's milk contains hormone residues that can contribute to female hormonal imbalance symptoms such as fibroid tumors, breast cysts, PMS and bloating because of the estrogenic effects. These residues also affect men as well. When I have a client who complains about being lactose-intolerant, I simply tell him or her to stop dairy products completely. In a matter of a few days, my client begins to feel much better and experiences less mucus production, sinus problems, stomach distress and allergy symptoms.

I have listed some nondairy options for you that are extremely nutritious. These natural substitutes can be found at most health food stores or supermarkets.

- Soy milk—lactose- and cholesterol-free
- Almond milk—lactose- and cholesterol-free
- Yogurt—dairy in origin, but culturing makes it a living food beneficial for health
- Soy cheese—lactose- and cholesterol-free
- Rice cheese—lactose- and cholesterol-free
- Rice milk—lactose- and cholesterol-free
- Tofu—supreme dairy replacement, made from soy bean, no cholesterol

It is true that milk is mentioned in the Bible. Milk was indeed common nourishment among the Israelites and, along with honey, symbolized good health!

> So I have come down to deliver them out of the hand of the Egyptians, and to bring them up from that land to a good and large land, to a land flowing with milk and honey.
> —Exodus 3:8, NKJV

Yes, the Bible clearly speaks about milk. Goat's milk, that is. There is a big difference between the milk of a cow and the milk of a goat.

And thou shalt have goats' milk enough for thy food, for the food of thy household, and for the maintenance of thy maidens.

—PROVERBS 27:27

Raw goat's milk is far superior to cow's milk. It is naturally homogeneous, has more quality protein and has a higher amount of niacin and thiamine. Thiamine is one of the most important of the B-complex vitamins involved in all of life's vital processes from the cradle to the grave. Besides being one of the cleanest of animals, goats are virtually free of all of the diseases that afflict cows. Goat's milk is not commonly used today in this country primarily because of economic reasons. Cows yield much larger quantities of milk than goats. It would take five hundred goats to produce the milk that one hundred cows can produce. Since the availability of raw goat's milk is scarce in our cosmopolitan society, I have chosen to recommend nondairy alternatives.

WHEAT

It's not what it's cracked up to be anymore.

For many generations wheat has been one of the main sources of protein, amino acids, complex carbohydrates and fiber. Approximately 360 million metric tons of wheat are harvested worldwide each year. These days, we do not get all of the benefits of wheat that generations long ago enjoyed. The reason is because wheat is now refined. During the refining process, wheat loses about 80 percent of vitamins B_1, B_2, B_3 and B_6; 98 percent of vitamin E; and 90 percent of minerals and micronutrients. In my opinion, refinement completely strips wheat of its God-designed benefits for our body. Since the advent of refinement, there has been an increase in the incidence of allergy food sensitivity or intolerance to wheat. As people are exposed more and more to refined, enzyme-depleted and processed foods, the body's ability to digest is weakened, and assimilation does not efficiently take place. This leaves large amounts of undigested material that the immune system treats as potentially toxic. The more toxic a body becomes, the more severe the food sensitivities become. The most common food intolerances that occur these days are to wheat, dairy products, sugar, yeast and coffee. This only confirms that, during this 90-day plan, eliminating these substances that block optimal health from your diet will be instrumental in achieving a higher level of immunity.

What are the symptoms of food allergies or sensitivities? You may experience one or more of the following symptoms after consuming an offending food: bloating, tiredness, nausea, racing pulse, palpitations, headache, anxiety, insomnia and sinus problems, to name a few.

I recommend that you make millet bread your bread of choice. Millet is a balanced, gluten-free grain. It is rich in amino acids, alkalizing to the stomach, and most importantly, great for people who are allergic or sensitive to wheat. In addition, millet is perfectly acceptable for people battling candida albicans yeast overgrowth syndrome. Many of my clients who have recurrent digestive complaints, which include gas, bloating, indigestion and discomfort, feel very well and have more energy after eliminating wheat from their diets. Sinus problems especially improve after both wheat and dairy are removed from the diet. Women tell me that they love the fact that their bloating disappears!

> Judah and the land of Israel were your traders. They traded for your merchandise wheat of Minnith, millet, honey, oil, and balm.
>
> —EZEKIEL 27:17, NKJV

CAFFEINE

Many people in this country depend on their morning cup of java to jump-start their engines. The coffee industry has blossomed into thousands of specialty coffee shops all across America. In any one of these shops, you can hear people ordering latte, ole, mocha, vanilla, raspberry and many more exotic concoctions. The one thing they all have in common is caffeine. Not only do these highly personalized coffee blends taste good, but they make you feel good. But alas, the feeling is only temporary. This is why you see these shops doing fabulously. The coffee industry knows that you'll be back for more. Why? Because coffee is an addictive stimulant. The caffeine in coffee, or soft drinks and iced tea for that matter, can cause jumpiness, anxiety, nerve problems and heart palpitations. So many of my clients used to consume four to eight cups of coffee per day—along with soda and iced tea! Many of these people were being treated by their family physicians for nervous disorders. Their physicians never even asked about their dietary habits, or these clients never thought to mention their high caffeine intake. Once you wean yourself off of caffeine, you give your body a chance to show you what good, pure energy feels like.

Other negative effects of excessive caffeine consumption are headaches, stomach and digestive problems, high blood pressure, irritability, mood swings, and too much acidity in the body that can result in disease. It leaches B vitamins from the body, especially thiamine, which is important for stress control. In addition, it depletes your body of essential minerals, especially calcium and potassium. Most importantly, caffeine taxes the adrenal glands to the point of exhaustion. This in turn can cause hormonal imbalances that can lead to dreadful symptoms, especially in women. In men, excessive caffeine can contribute to prostate problems. Excessive caffeine use has been implicated in PMS, bladder problems and blood sugar problems, including diabetes and hypoglycemia.

Along with the negative effects on the body, caffeine can be of benefit in small to moderate amounts. If you suffer from any anxiety-related condition, I suggest you steer completely away from caffeine. If you are not an anxious type-A personality, that is, a high goal-oriented, perfectionist type, you may use caffeine occasionally in small amounts. Moderate amounts of caffeine have been used for centuries for its therapeutic benefit. These benefits include weight control, opening of the breathing passages in asthmatics, overcoming fatigue, increased capacity for intellectual tasks and decreased drowsiness.

Caffeine also has analgesic properties. Aspirin preparations contain caffeine. Many people know that if you take an aspirin with a drink containing caffeine, the pain relief will be enhanced. Caffeine can cause thermogenesis, or calorie burning. This can be an aid to obese people whose metabolism needs a boost. The amount of caffeine in one cup of coffee can boost the metabolic rate for about two to three hours. So you see, in moderate amounts, caffeine can be an aid to us in our daily lives. Unfortunately, many people are out of control these days. Caffeine and sugar are the fuel that keeps many men and women functioning in this fast-paced world. You must make a conscious choice about caffeine consumption. If you are going to build your immune system, I don't believe in putting something into your body that is addictive, a mineral leacher or a glandular system zapper. There are natural alternatives to help wean you off caffeine. This must be done slowly, though, because you will have withdrawal symptoms.

You may substitute coffee with herbal teas sweetened with stevia extract. I especially like roasted dandelion tea. It has a faint coffee taste that is reminiscent of the real thing. Other choices are carob instead of chocolate and herbal energy supplements that do not contain mahuang, which is another addictive stimulant. A small amount of caffeine for therapeutic benefit can be derived from drinking a cup of green tea. Do not consume it before bed, however, because you may not be able to fall off to sleep.

> Whether therefore ye eat, or drink, or whatsoever
> ye do, do all to the glory of God.
> —1 CORINTHIANS 10:31

No caffeine? Now what?

The supplements recommended on the first 30 days will prepare you to eliminate caffeine.

Instead of sodas that contain caffeine and sugar, add to seltzer water or club soda a quarter cup of unsweetened fruit juice, or simply add a slice of lime, lemon or orange. Instead of coffee, drink herbal teas sweetened with stevia extract, or drink Postum or Pero coffee, which are substitutes available at health food stores. Instead of chocolate, try carob.

ALCOHOL

Alcohol is another substance that, with excessive use, has a negative impact on health. When used in moderation, naturally fermented wine is more than just an alcoholic beverage. Being naturally fermented means that it can aid the body like yogurt and other fermented foods. There are still small, family-owned and operated wineries that make wines free of additives and chemicals.

Wine contains many important nutrients, which include magnesium, iron, calcium, potassium and phosphorus. In addition, wine contains highly absorbable B vitamins. Wine, in moderation, acts as a sedative for the heart, arteries and blood pressure. A glass or two of white wine with dinner has been shown in some studies to cut the risk of heart disease by 50 percent. Wine relieves nervous tension and stress, frees the circulation and reduces pain. These are the health benefits of moderate wine consumption.

Yet you'll find very few doctors who recommend wine to their patients—and here's why. Excessive alcohol consumption can lead to dependency or addiction. The serious conditions related to alcohol dependency or addiction include liver degeneration and disease, nervousness, short-term memory loss, blood sugar imbalances, mineral deficiency, mood swings, anger, aggressive behavior and depression. Excessive alcohol intake brings about degeneration in the body and has absolutely no place in an immune-boosting program. A little wine with dinner is not strictly prohibited (after 90 days) if you are so inclined. Just remember: Moderation is the key. But I'd like to suggest a better way: Drink grape juice. Concord grape juice has all of the nutrients, but none of the negatives of alcohol. Grape juice includes grape seeds–and grape seed extract is a powerful anti-oxidant.

> Do not mix with winebibbers, or with gluttonous eaters of meat; for the drunkard and the glutton will come to poverty, and drowsiness will clothe a man with rags.
>
> —PROVERBS 23:20–21, NKJV

SMOKING

Everyone knows that smoking is hazardous to your health. After all, we are living in the information age. And since we are, let me give you a little more information about smoking that you may not be aware of. Smoking is the largest single preventable cause of illness and premature death in the United States. It is connected to chronic bronchitis, emphysema and cancers of the lung, larynx, pharynx, mouth, esophagus, pancreas and bladder. There is also a connection linking smoking during pregnancy with complications and retarded fetal development. In addition, smoking ages you. According to the Canadian Cancer Society, a one-pack-a-day smoker is at age fifty physically as old as a nonsmoker at age fifty-eight!

My own father was a smoker. I can remember him going for a bicycle ride after dinner while smoking a cigarette! You should know my father suffered from heart disease, emphysema and cancer. Needless to say, I have never smoked a cigarette and never will! For those who smoke, the health hazards of smoking are numerous, including endangering your loved ones, especially children, because of the dangerous effect of secondhand smoke. You are predisposing your family or coworkers to respiratory illness or possibly nicotine-related cancer. If you do not stop smoking for yourself, then do it for those around you. It is a dangerous, expensive and dirty habit that stains your hands and teeth and fouls your breath. It pollutes your home, car and workplace. Before your smoking habit kills you, kill your smoking habit.

That's easier said than done. Since I am not a smoker, you might be thinking, *That's easy for her to say.* I realize that quitting the smoking habit can be one of the hardest tasks you ever undertake. If you are ready, I have a plan to help you kick the habit and reverse the damage that has already occurred. That's the good news. It is encouraging to know that almost all of smoking's health hazards can be totally reversed once you stop. Here is how the plan works. First, begin on the weekend, ideally on Saturday. Try to begin this plan when you are on a regular schedule—a relatively calm time of the year away from parties, birthdays, tax time and so forth, but do not begin while on vacation or under unusual stress from your job. Mark a goal on your calendar, and label it Smoke Free! Begin to work toward that goal. I have found that the fourteen-day plan works for most of my clients, while some people can achieve their smoke-free day sooner. The longer you drag it out, the longer it will be before your body begins to reverse smoking's negative effects.

During the first seven days, follow the makeover eating plan. Take 200 micrograms of chromium. (If you are over 150 pounds, you may take 400 micrograms). Chromium will help to balance your blood sugar, thereby lessening any symptoms of withdrawal. Cut down on the number of cigarettes you smoke this week by one-half. If you feel the urge to smoke, just chew gum or munch on carrot or celery sticks to satisfy the feeling of having something in your mouth. Get rid of all lighters and matches. Tell your family, friends and coworkers that you are giving up this health-destroying habit, and enlist their support.

As you approach the eighth day, cut down your smoking by one-half once again. The majority of people experience withdrawal symptoms, though some do not, ranging from very mild to very difficult. Withdrawal can best be described by the following symptoms: headache, tiredness, cough, nervousness, dizziness, constipation, sore throat and craving for a cigarette. To help minimize these symptoms, try exercising, sleeping more at night, drinking plenty of water and eating a lot of fresh fruit to even out the release of nicotine from the body. If you are constipated, slowly add fiber into the diet, and this problem should pass quickly. Just be patient and ride out these symptoms. They will pass.

On days ten through thirteen continue to cut back on your cigarettes by one-half each day. By day fourteen you should be smoke free! Now that you have accomplished this milestone, ask God to continue to give you strength to move forward, never back. Cigarette smoking is now in your past. Take a deep breath and know that every breath you take from this moment on is helping to regenerate your entire body. Stay on the chromium; it will help you conquer any unhealthy craving, whether it be cigarettes, sugar or alcohol.

After you break the smoking habit, get your car cleaned and detailed to rid it of the smell of smoke. Clean your house from top to bottom—wash drapes and rugs; wash down walls and counters; throw away ash trays. Keep chewing gum handy when you're under stress, and remember how wonderful it is to be set free from smoking.

SALT

Many people believe that salt contributes to high blood pressure, kidney problems, migraines and fluid retention. This is true when you consume salt in excessive amounts. The truth is that salt is very important for body balance. I have some clients who come to see me for a health-building program that brag about never eating salt. They are very surprised when I tell them that salt is needed for proper body chemistry. Adequate sodium is needed for strong blood, healthy organs and glands, nutrient transportation and blood pressure.

Blood pressure? That's right. We traditionally hear that salt is responsible for increasing blood pressure. I personally have suffered from low blood pressure and was proud of the fact that I never salted my food or ate salty foods. Then I learned that while I was right about table salt being almost totally devoid of nutritional value, our bodies require good, healthy salt that is highly absorbable and useable. Too little salt can lead to lack of vitality, stagnated blood and foggy thinking. When I added salt to my diet, my blood pressure became stable, and I felt stronger and more vital. This is not a license to overdo it (remember, everything in moderation)! Low salt, not no salt, is the way to go. I particularly like Bragg's Liquid Aminos as a healthful way to add sodium to your diet. It has one-tenth the sodium of table salt, sixteen amino acids and is made from water and soybeans. It tastes wonderful.

Other good ways to receive healthy salt for your system are olives, pickles and sea salt.

GREEN SUPERFOODS

It has been said that eating green superfoods is almost like receiving a little transfusion to enhance immunity and promote energy and well-being. They are one of the richest sources of essential nutrients. Nutritionally they are more compact, concentrated and potent than regular greens like salads and green vegetables. In addition, green superfoods are purposely grown and harvested to maximize and insure high vitamin, mineral and amino acid concentrations. The following are green superfoods that are available in most health food stores across the country.

Blue and blue-green algae are the most potent forms of beta carotene available in the world. These are the perfect superfoods because they are brimming with superior quality proteins, fiber, vitamins, minerals and enzymes.

Spirulina is an algae that is extremely high in protein and rich in B vitamins, amino acids, beta carotene and essential fatty acids. Easy to digest, it boosts energy quickly and sustains it for long periods of time.

Barley grass contains minerals, proteins, enzymes and chlorophyll. It contains more vitamin C, vitamin

B$_{12}$ and calcium than cow's milk. It also helps inflammatory conditions of the stomach and digestive system.

Wheatgrass has been used around the world for many serious diseases to rebuild, cleanse, and strengthen the body because of its incredible nutritional value. Fifteen pounds of wheat grass is equivalent to almost four hundred pounds of the most perfectly grown vegetables.

Kyo-Green is my all-time favorite green superfood because of the synergism of the combination of ingredients. Kyo-Green contains barley, wheatgrass, chlorella and kelp. This is a potent formula that helps to cleanse the bloodstream, to detoxify the system and to supply the body with minerals, enzymes and many important nutrient-providing energy for enhanced daily performance. I personally use Kyo-Green powder every day. These ingredients do so much more for your body than any of the green superfoods alone. I recommend that you use this on your immune makeover eating plan because of the wonderful formulation of ingredients. Try it and feel the difference.

POWER MUSHROOMS

In my quest for wellness, I used what I call power mushrooms. Now the interest in these same mushrooms has literally...mushroomed. Researchers have found that certain types of mushrooms are filled with a grocery list of substances that may help in fighting disease. Most exciting is that they boost immunity, and some may even be effective against cancer and heart disease. Researchers have also discovered that mushrooms produce many beneficial compounds that help their survival against other fungi and microbes, and these same substances can help humans as well. Mushrooms contain compounds known as polysaccharides, which spark the immune system by helping the body create T cells, which, as you remember, are immune system warriors that destroy invaders and may halt tumor growth.

It is thought that incorporating any of the power mushrooms into your diet will result in dramatic health recoveries because of the synergism with the immune system. According to author Christopher Hobbs in his book *Medicinal Mushrooms*, the chemicals, steroids and terpenes that mushrooms also contain are thought to help fight the formation of cancerous tumors. By adding one of these power mushrooms to your immune-boosting eating plan, you will be adding one more powerful weapon to your immune army. Here are three main power mushrooms—wonderful immune boosters from God's bounty:

Reishi—stimulates immunity and has antitumor properties. It is anti-inflammatory, and it helps to alleviate arthritis.

Shiitake—has possible antiviral and anticancer properties, and is an energizer. It is also delicious when used in cooking. In the immune-boosting recipe section, you will find wonderful recipes that use this flavorful health-boosting mushroom.

Maitake—has antitumor properties. It may protect the liver and lower blood pressure. It contains beta glucans, which are chemicals that boost immunity.

ANTIOXIDANTS

We know that our immune protection consists of

macrophages, white blood cells, antibodies, lymphatic tissue and the thymus gland. In recent years, science has uncovered health-destroying substances called free radicals that attack the body's defenses, weakening and damaging healthy cells so that they will not properly protect us.

There are three basic sources of free radical activity. First, free radicals are formed as by-products during exercise, illness and by taking certain medications. Second is air pollution, smoke, excessive sun exposure, radiation and pesticides. And third, free radicals form other free radicals. Increased free radical production is linked to many ailments, including accelerated aging, cancer, heart disease, arthritis, Alzheimer's disease and even AIDS.

Antioxidants come to the rescue! Antioxidants are a group of vitamins, minerals and other substances that neutralize free radicals, thereby preventing the weakening and damaging of our cells. Their job is to travel the bloodstream and localize in our cells and organs and neutralize free radicals. After they neutralize or quench these free radicals, they become inactive and are eliminated from the body. This means we continually need to supply our bodies either through diet or supplementation or both.

The four major antioxidants are pro-vitamin A (or beta carotene), vitamin C, vitamin E and selenium. These four antioxidant nutrients provide a four-point attack. Pro-vitamin A, or beta carotene, quenches singlet oxygen molecules. Vitamin C protects tissues and blood components, while vitamin E protects cell membranes; selenium is a vital part of antioxidant enzymes.

All together, these powerful four "mop up" free radicals as they form and before they do damage to our systems. I personally use and recommend Carlson ACES as my formula of choice for antioxidant protection. Their formula contains 10,000 International Units pro-vitamin A (or beta carotene), 1,000 milligrams of vitamin C in a non-acidic calcium ascorbate form, 400 International Units of vitamin E in the form of natural d-alpha tocopherol and 100 micrograms of selenium. The dose is two soft gel capsules daily.

Science does agree: Have a cup of tea

For thousands of years, people of Japan and China have relied on tea to cure a multitude of ailments and to prevent disease. Now, science is in agreement with what these people have always known.

What science has found that is so exciting and significant is that tea, primarily green and black, contains health-promoting antioxidants that will prevent free-radical damage, avert some of the effects of aging, stimulate our immune system to help fight existing disease and boost its ability to protect the body from viral and bacterial invaders, allergies, cancer, arthritis, heart disease and stroke. Scientists are particularly excited about green tea, which, in addition to being a rich source of antioxidants, appears to increase the activity of other antioxidant enzymes within the body. It also contains other valuable substances called catechins, polyphenols, flavonoids and proanthocyanidins, which make green tea extremely effective in fighting heart disease, stroke and cancer.

This is not to minimize the wonderful properties of

black tea. In addition to helping to prevent and dissolve blood clots, black tea also appears to protect the arteries from narrowing and becoming clogged by cholesterol. Research from the National Institute of Nutrition in Rome revealed that drinking green tea can increase antioxidant activity in your blood by almost 50 percent in just thirty minutes, and black tea can do the same in fifty minutes. In both cases, the effect lasted for almost ninety minutes. Other studies have confirmed that drinking green tea can prevent some forms of cancer, including cancer of the stomach, small intestine, pancreas, colon, lungs and breast cancer.

So, for those of you who need scientific proof, we now have it. God made these substances to promote health and to keep us well even before science had to prove it to us. God truly provided everything we need in nature to keep us healthy. He has and will always be way ahead of us. He knew that we would need antioxidant protection now more than ever. Now science agrees with this knowledge that we can truly prosper and be in health. (See 3 John 2.)

IMMUNE-BOOSTING OLIVE OIL

When olive oil is used in your diet, it stimulates metabolism, promotes digestion and lubricates mucous membranes. In addition, the vitamin E in olive oil is an antioxidant. The monounsaturated fatty acids in olive oil help to lower LDL, or "bad" cholesterol, levels without affecting HDL, or "good" cholesterol, or triglyceride levels. On your immune-boosting eating plan, you will be using olive oil to cook with and as a dressing for your salads. Use olive oil that is labeled "extra-virgin." This guarantees that the oil has been cold pressed from freshly harvested olives and does not contain chemicals. Extra-virgin olive oil supplies the best flavor, and oil that is golden yellow in color is of higher quality than green. Whenever you cook, use olive oil. Use olive oil also in salad dressings, vegetables and in making sandwiches. It is interesting to note that in countries where olive oil is consumed extensively, such as Greece, Italy and Spain, there is a low incidence of cardiovascular diseases.

While I consider olive oil to be the best in food preparation, here are other oils that contribute to optimal health: canola, almond, flaxseed, safflower, walnut and sesame. If you do not like the taste of olive oil, canola oil is a good alternative because it is high in monounsaturated fats and helps prevent heart disease just as olive oil does. Now that you know the best oils, here are the ones to stay away from: coconut, peanut, cottonseed, palm and palm kernel oil. Please take the time to read food labels, as these oils are commonly used in many processed foods. If you are following the 90-Day Immune System Makeover eating plan, these oils will not be anywhere near your body. So avoiding them will not be a problem.

THE EATING PLAN

Use the 90-Day Immune System Makeover eating plan with detoxification. It is high in nutrition, and it eliminates foods that can lower the immune response (white sugar, white flour, dairy products, wheat and yeast). In addition, there is emphasis on blood sugar balancing.

On rising:
- 8-ounce glass of water with ½ fresh lemon to clean kidneys; add stevia extract to sweeten. If there is flatulence, add 1 teaspoon of apple cider vinegar.

Breakfast—have one of the following:
- 1 or 2 poached or hard-boiled eggs on a slice of millet bread
- Oatmeal (or oat bran) with 1 tablespoon Bragg's Liquid Aminos
- Buckwheat pancakes with a little butter or almond butter
- Millet toast with almond butter

Midmorning—have one of the following:
- A green drink (Kyo-Green or liquid chlorophyll)
- A cup of dandelion tea
- A small bottle of water

Lunch—have one of the following:
- A fresh green salad with lemon and olive oil dressing
- An open-face millet sandwich with mayonnaise, veggies, seafood, turkey or chicken
- Vegetable soup with a piece of millet bread
- Chicken, tuna or vegetable pasta salad

Midafternoon—have one of the following with a cup of green tea with stevia:
- Rice crackers or baked corn chips with rice cheese or soy cheese
- A bottle of water with a hard-boiled or deviled egg
- Raw veggies (if tolerated)

Dinner—have one of the following:
- Baked, broiled or poached fish or chicken with steamed brown rice
- Baked potato with Bragg's Liquid Aminos or rice cheese
- Oriental stir-fry with brown rice
- Small omelet with a veggie filling
- Vegetarian casserole
- Hot or cold vegetable pasta salad

Before bed:
- Have a cup of herb tea such as dandelion or chamomile; add stevia to sweeten and balance blood sugar.

1. *Kyo-Green:* A complete green superfood that contains protein and all the B vitamins. It heals the intestinal tract, strengthens the liver and boosts immune health. It is a good detoxifier and blood cleanser rich in chlorophyll.
2. *Stevia extract:* Designed to aid in blood sugar balance, even in cases of severe sugar imbalance. Stevia is twenty-five times sweeter than sugar. It also has zero calories. Health-related benefits include those associated with regulating blood sugar, lowering blood pressure and even preventing tooth decay. *Stevia Rebaudiana,* a South American sweetening leaf, is also antifungal and antibacterial. Stevia has been used for hundreds of years in countries such as Paraguay and Japan as an important dietary supplement. Simply adding a few drops of stevia as a dietary supplement to your food and beverages is a wonderful way to make it a part of your healthful lifestyle. Make a delicious lemonade with fresh lemons, water and stevia extract. Drink it throughout the day. It tastes great and helps keep blood sugar stable—enjoy!
3. *Bragg's Amino Acids:* A natural health alternative to soy sauce made from soybean and purified water. Spray or dash liquid aminos on salads and dressings, soups, veggies, rice and beans, tofu, wok and stir-frys, macrobiotics, casseroles, potatoes, meats, fish, poultry, jerky, tempeh, gravies and sauces and popcorn. It contains no chemicals, no alcohol, no additives, no preservatives, no added sodium, no coloring agents and no wheat; it is not fermented and is an excellent plant protein.
4. *ACES+Zinc: Vitamins A, C, E and selenium.* These antioxidants neutralize highly reactive molecules. Air pollution, tobacco smoke and ozone, as well as pesticides, dietary fats and heavy exercise, can produce unstable substances in the body called free radicals. Research has established that excess free radicals can damage healthy cells. Our bodies naturally suppress free radicals with these vitamins and minerals.
5. *Maitake/power mushroom:* Powerful compound for enhancing healthy defense system mechanism. It promotes proper lipid metabolism in the liver and healthy levels of cholesterol.
6. *B-complex with pantothenic acid:* Essential for proper functioning of the nervous system and perhaps the most important nutritional factor for healthy nerve cells. It plays a role in conversion of carbohydrates into energy, the metabolism of fats and protein and the maintenance of muscle tone in the GI tract, and it supports the integrity of the skin, hair and liver.

EXERCISE

Move it so you won't lose it! During these first 30 days, you will begin a transformation. You are making lifestyle changes that will benefit the immunity of your body as well as your mind and spirit. While you detoxify your body during this first phase, you will be following a plan of eating that eliminates all of the substances that lower immunity. You will also incorporate exercise into your life. We have become so used to modern conveniences that do our work for us—for example, vacuum cleaners, electric mixers, washing machines and dryers. I can remember my grandmother beating the dust out of her rugs with a broom and then using that broom to sweep the entire house afterward. Later in the day, she would wash her clothes by hand with a wash board and basin and carry the clothes out to the backyard to hang on the clothesline. If there was time left in the day, she managed to wax the floor. In addition, I can remember the sound and smell of my grandmother making her own bread dough, kneading it by hand over and over and then baking it to perfection.

Think about this for a moment. This woman gave herself a workout every day just by doing her daily chores. She experienced a tiredness at the end of the day that felt wonderful because as she used to tell me, it was a "good tired." It was the kind that gives you a restful sleep. I often remember my grandmother's words, and I love that "good tired" feeling myself. It's the kind that comes when your muscles have been worked, your legs have been stretched, your arms have lifted, pushed and pulled, your waist has been twisted and bent and your back has lifted and extended. Everything these days is so automatic that cleaning the house or anything else just is not enough to make us "good tired." Without enough movement each day, your stress continues to be stored in your muscles. Breathing becomes shallow, you become irritable, headaches become a daily occurrence, and short tempers flair. No wonder so many people are suffering from stress-related illness. Exercise not only to relieve stress and improve your cardiovascular health, but to experience being "good tired."

Exercise aids detoxification. It helps you eliminate toxins faster. During the first 30 days, I recommend that you begin a walking program. Start first with a 30-minute walk. If you walk alone, you can have time to yourself to think or de-stress and enjoy the scenery. You may want to walk with a friend because time seems to fly, and it gives you a chance to share and use each other as a sounding board. I personally do both. There are times when I want time to myself to be with God as I walk. Then there are times that a walking buddy is good medicine when faced with a problem. This way you de-stress as you get advice from someone who really cares about you. I have found that most problems seem not so important after a brisk walk or workout.

If, however, you are not able to walk at this point because of illness or handicap, try to make some type of exercise part of your daily plan. Start slow with one- to three-pound weights and do some biceps or triceps curls, ride a bike, walk a treadmill, swim, take a water aerobics class, a stretching class or anything to get your body moving!

An exercise program you can stick with

According to the Center for Disease Control and Prevention, only about 15 percent of American adults work out three or more times a week. In addition, over half of the people who start an exercise program wind up quitting within six months of when they started, most often within the first three months. I believe this is because of the approach that most people take when beginning an exercise program. It does not have to be a painful, frustrating experience. If you are over age forty-five, have not had a checkup in the past two years or suffer from diabetes, heart disease, high blood pressure or other chronic illnesses, see your physician before beginning an exercise program.

During this first 30 days you are going to incorporate exercise into your life. You can do this very easily by building in motivators that will insure long-term, lifestyle-changing success.

First, get yourself a calendar dedicated just to your exercise routine. Mark off one month at a time, and plan to work out around the same time of the day on the same days of each week. (For example, Monday, Wednesday and Friday at nine o'clock in the morning for thirty minutes.) Each time you exercise, record on your exercise calendar the type of exercise and the actual length. This will encourage you and give you a sense of accomplishment. As the weeks pass, you will notice how your strength, flexibility and energy have increased. After a month or two, change your routine by changing locations or activity. For example, ride a bike instead of walking, or do both during the week or add light weight training. The more you make exercise a part of your life, the less stress, fatigue and excuses you will have for not exercising for optimal health. It is really true—if you don't move it, you will lose it when it comes to optimal health.

Warm up for five to ten minutes by stretching or doing light calisthenics. Cool down after your workout—walk around slowly until your heart rate slows down and returns to normal. Stopping suddenly can be dangerous, particularly if you are elderly. Finish your workout by stretching slowly; do not bounce or stretch beyond your limits, or you could injure yourself. Drink water to avoid dehydration; do not wait to feel thirsty. Drink before, during and after exercise to keep yourself adequately hydrated.

Choose the exercise that best suits your current health status.

To get the therapeutic benefits of exercise, find a regimen proven to work against what you're battling in your current health condition. It should be one that will give you enough of a mental and physical boost to keep you coming back for more. According to the American College of Sports Medicine, the following are the five most common ailments that plague Americans today. As always, consult your physician before embarking on a new exercise program. This is especially true if you suffer from any of these conditions.

Diabetes affects over eight million people in our country. The best form of exercise is daily walking, running, biking or other forms of aerobic exercise. The more vigorous the better. Benefits include greater control of blood sugar for insulin-dependent diabetics, though exercise needs to be coordinated with insulin shots and meals. Type two diabetics can experience weight loss, which can result in a reduction of medication. Some people may be able to eliminate the need to take insulin entirely.

Weightlifting, along with group aerobic and weight workouts, seems to work best for *depression*. This is especially true for women because of the improvement in self-image. Over time, regular exercise relieves symptoms in many, if not all, sufferers.

Daily stretching and low-impact aerobic exercise, like walking or swimming, plus two or three weekly sessions of strength training work best for *arthritis* sufferers, who number over thirty-three million in our country. The benefits are less pain and more freedom of movement. Take care not to overexert yourself, or you may experience back pain or spinal cord compression.

High blood pressure responds best to moderate aerobic exercise at a pace that allows you to have a conversation. Weight training is allowed for those who have their pressure under control with medication. Most hypertensive people can expect a ten to fifteen point drop in their blood pressure in about four months. Often this is enough to eliminate the need to take medication for lowering blood pressure. You must be consistent, however, because blood pressure tends to rise if you give up your exercise program.

Helpful for *osteoporosis* is lifting weights two or three times weekly, focusing on arms and legs. Many women can expect a halt in bone loss and may even rebuild bone.

AFTER EXERCISE LAVENDER-MINT BATH

This wonderful bath is soothing to your muscles as well as your mind. Pour into your warm bath water:

- 2 Tbsp. peppermint oil
- 2 Tbsp. spearmint oil
- 2 Tbsp. lavender oil

- For detoxifying bath: 1 bag sea salt and 1 box baking soda

Relax and enjoy! After exercise, you will look forward to this bath. Use it as a reward for being diligent in following your exercise plan.

WHAT TO EXPECT

One of the most important and often misunderstood areas in the strengthening and rebuilding of your body is the symptoms and changes that follow the beginning of a better nutritional program. During these first 30 days as you introduce foods of higher quality while eliminating lower quality foods and toxic substances such as coffee, tea, chocolate, tobacco, excess salt and alcohol, remarkable things begin to happen to the body as well as the mind. When you first eliminate lower-grade foods and introduce superior foods, alive and more natural than you are accustomed to, a headache of letdown occurs. This letdown usually lasts about forty-eight hours, followed by a feeling of well-being and strength.

During this entire 90-Day Immune System Makeover your body will begin to discard the lower-grade materials to make room for new superior materials that are now being consumed. The body will use them to make new and healthier tissue. This is God's plan for us. He made our bodies to produce health unless our interference is too great. Notice the self-curing nature of many conditions such as colds, fevers, cuts, swellings and bruises. These are examples of how the body always strives for health and healing unless we do something to stop the process.

When you begin the makeover program, you will be detoxifying your system. Please give your system a chance to adjust and complete this very important first phase. Symptoms may occur as you detoxify, improve your diet and eliminate the health robbers (caffeine, sugar, alcohol).

During this initial phase, energy in the external parts of your body, such as the muscles and skin, moves to the vital internal organs to start the regeneration and reconstruction process. This shunting of much of the power to the internal region produces a feeling of less energy in the muscles, which the mind interprets as weakness. In actuality the power is increased, but most of it is being used for rebuilding the important organs, and less energy is used for the muscles. But be assured that this is not true weakness—only a redeploying of energy to more important internal parts. During this crucial phase it is important to rest and sleep more. This way even more energy can be used for regeneration. When you experience this, do not resort to any stimulant of any kind. This will defeat and stop the regeneration process.

It is important to have faith and patience. After a while, you will gain increasing strength, which will far exceed what you felt before you began this makeover program. Your degree of improvement hinges upon the correct understanding of this point. During this phase, rest and relax, limit social obligations and take it easy at work until it passes.

As you continue with the makeover, your body will gain more and more energy due to the wonderful live foods you are consuming in addition to the immune-boosting supplements. As your body builds energy, the more symptoms you may have. This is because energy is being used to discard toxic wastes, cellular debris and poisons. Realize that your body is becoming younger and healthier every day because you are throwing off more and more wastes that eventually would have brought pain, disease and much suffering.

I have found that those who have the most bothersome symptoms and follow through to their successful termination are avoiding some of the worst diseases that would certainly have developed if they had continued their same unhealthy lifestyle.

Your body is cyclical in nature, and health will be rebuilt in a series of gradual cycles. You will have good days and not-so-good days as you journey toward optimal immunity. You will feel better. Then a set of symptoms will occur, and you won't feel as well for a couple of days. Then you will recover and feel even better than before. And so it goes, each set of symptoms gradually becoming milder than the previous set because your body is becoming purer and less toxic each day. Your periods of feeling very well will become longer and longer and your "symptom days" less and less until you become relatively disease free.

Your body will be clean, your diet optimal and you will be taking proper immune supplementation. Continue to focus on God as your source for healing. Have faith, and watch this process. Before your very eyes you will see and feel signs that will cause you to be in awe of God's intelligence at work in your body, mind and spirit.

SUMMARY—YOUR IMMUNITY: WHAT CAN GO WRONG?

- *Poor diet:* Consumption of refined sugar can interfere with immunity. According to the *American Journal of Clinical Nutrition,* a study found that sugar slowed the ability of the immune system to eradicate, engulf and consume alien material. Sugar's effect on insulin levels restricts vitamin C's role in allowing immune cells to travel and destroy invaders in our body.

- *Lack of sleep:* Regeneration takes place while you sleep, rebuilding processes during sleep that do not take place during waking hours. Sleep experts agree that while seven hours of sleep per night is the minimum amount needed for a properly functioning immune system, eight hours is still optimal.

- *Alcohol:* It lowers immunity by inhibiting the ability of your white cells to react to infections.

- *Stress:* A study done in 1977 showed that blood taken from widows and widowers who were in the grieving process had reduced natural killer cell activity. Stress and a depressed mental out-look can lower immunity.

- *Overweight:* According to the *American Journal of Clinical Nutrition,* eating a low-fat diet may help boost the activity of your natural killer cells, thereby enhancing your immune response.

SHOPPING LIST FOR FIRST 30 DAYS

The following are available at almost any health food store.

- Stevia extract—liquid or powder
- Dandelion tea
- Rice cheese
- Rice or soy milk
- Brown rice
- ACES+Zinc—antioxidants
- Nature's Secret Ultimate Cleanse—detox
- B-complex with pantothenic acid
- Maitake power mushroom
- Kyo-Green—a green drink
- Green tea—decaffeinated
- Soy cheese
- Almond butter
- Bragg's Liquid Aminos
- Millet bread

For detoxifying bath: 1 bag sea salt and 1 box baking soda

PART TWO:

The Next 60 Days

The Next
60 Days

As we embark on this next phase, we are going to address sleep, yeast eradication, the importance of enzyme therapy, adrenal health and stress management. During this phase you will be very busy working to eliminate yeast and strengthening your glandular system. You will still be following the same eating plan as for the first 30 days. The only difference is that now you are moving up in the program to a rebalancing, regenerating phase. This is possible because during the first 30 days you have removed toxins, debris and lifestyle habits that in the past have prevented the regeneration process.

Immune System on the Blink? Think Zinc!

The health of your immune system is dependent to a large degree on the health of your thymus gland. Zinc, along with vitamins B_6 and C, is necessary for the

79

production of your thymic hormones. T cells, which are produced in your thymus gland, get a real boost from zinc. Zinc increases the number of circulating T cells in young and old alike. As we age, our chances of a zinc deficiency increase, and along with it, our thymus function suffers. It may even come to a halt! Zinc should be included in any program that builds the immune system because of the important role it plays in nourishing the thymus gland as well as liberating vitamin A from our liver. Vitamin A is another source of nourishment for our thymus gland.

When it comes to immunity, the health of your thymus gland is vitally important to immune defense. The thymus gland is located in the upper part of the chest behind the breast bone. It is a nursery for immune system cells that help fight infection. Unfortunately, as we grow older, this gland shrinks, and so does its effectiveness. Practitioners of natural medicine recommend the following exercise to stimulate the thymus gland, thereby boosting your immune health. Every morning tap the middle of the breastbone with your fingers for five minutes. That's all there is to it!

ACHIEVING AND MAINTAINING YOUR IDEAL WEIGHT

While it is true that weight loss is a natural result as you follow the 90-Day Immune Makeover, we still must cover this subject. Weight control, just like high immunity, should be a lifelong program. The word *calorie* is not a dirty word, except when you pile calories on. According to the American Council on Science and Health, a Big Mac has 563 calories, a

80

Whopper with cheese has 740 calories, a Taco Bell burrito has 466, two pieces of extra-crispy Kentucky Fried Chicken have 544 calories and a chocolate milk shake has 383 calories.

Calories are fuel for our bodies. Just as the quality of the fuel you put in your car's engine determines its performance, so the quality of food determines your body's performance. The amount of fuel your body needs varies at different stages in your life. If you have teenagers at home, you know by your grocery bills that massive quantities of calories are being consumed by these active young adults.

As we age, however, our caloric needs begin to taper off. A man at age fifty-one can get along on 90 percent of the number of calories he needed twenty-five years before. But remember, while caloric needs are less, the quality of food needs to remain high. Ideally, the number of calories we consume should approximately match the number we need to keep our bodies in proper working order.

In the new millennium, this is easier said than done. We are surrounded by rich and tempting foods with no will power to resist them. Consequently, most Americans take in more calories than they burn off. When we don't burn off the excess calories, our bodies simply store them. Like a well thought-out machine, our body has a fuel storage and/or reserve tank. These are known as the fat cells. With continued overconsumption of high-calorie foods, fat cells will expand almost limitlessly to store away fat. That is, if we don't exercise to burn it off beforehand. Therefore, the easiest, most efficient way to reach and maintain your ideal weight is to tackle both sides of the equation at once. Reduce the amount of fuel or calories you take in daily, while at the same time increase the work or exercise you do each day. This two-pronged attack will bring your weight into a healthy, immune-boosting, life-sustaining balance.

On the immune-makeover eating plan, we do not count calories, but we do make sure that we are eating healthy and with balance. This will discourage you from overeating. In time you will no longer crave lower quality foods that are high in calories and low in quality nutrition. As you eat with balance and incorporate some forms of activity or exercise each day, your body will begin to shed weight if it needs to or gain weight if that's what you need. Again, we are giving the body what it needs to become strong and balanced. Allow your body to experience balance. This is our natural state of being. This is the way God intended us to be.

As you follow the 90-Day Immune System Makeover, there are a few simple tips to keep in mind to help you burn off fat to protect your heart, lower your blood pressure and improve your cholesterol levels. First of all, walk instead of drive whenever you can. Park in the area of the parking lot farthest from your destination and walk. Get off the elevator one floor early and walk upstairs. Go to a shopping mall and walk, walk, walk. Use small plates and fill them up instead of large ones that can look half filled, tempting you to pile on more food. Eat slowly. Never eat alone, and do not buy snacks to have on hand in case guests drop in. Shop for your groceries after you eat so you won't make impulsive hunger-driven food purchases, which are usually unhealthy in nature.

When you carry extra weight, the chance of serious health problems escalates. Hypertension is twice as common among obese persons, and diabetes is four times as prevalent. Obese persons are three times more likely to have heart attacks. In the case of hypertension and heart disease, it is believed that the heart must work harder to pump blood in order to provide an adequate supply to the rest of the body. As far as diabetes goes, it seems that additional fat cells place too great a demand on the amount of insulin, thus glucose levels accumulate dangerously in the blood. For your health's sake and for optimal immunity, it is wise to use these 90 days as an opportunity to really "go for it." All the tools you will need are contained in this book. Just apply the principles, and you will see results not only where your weight is concerned, but also in every area of your life.

Weight loss is not the focus of this makeover; balance is. If you are in balance, then you will not be overweight! This is not a diet; it is a plan for life, health and service. Despite all of the books and articles, there is no such thing as a miracle diet that will quickly melt away pounds and keep them off. Just like weight gain was a gradual process, achieving your ideal weight is a lifelong process. It is something you gradually scale down to.

There are three basic elements to consider when trying to arrive at your ideal weight: patience, perseverance and psychological support from family and friends.

SLEEP

Studies show that people with sleep difficulties or people who don't get enough sleep have fewer natural killer cells, therefore increasing susceptibility to disease. In addition, lack of sleep can wreak havoc with the immune system. During sleep, your body is hard at work repairing, rebuilding and regenerating your system. Without proper sleep, your body doesn't get a chance to take care of you!

You are at the 60-day mark now, and sleep is crucial. You have begun the rebuilding phase of the immune system makeover program.

TIPS FOR SLEEPING

- Establish a routine. Synchronize your sleep/wake cycle.
- Eliminate coffee, tea, sodas, and chocolate. If you must drink coffee, have it six hours before bed.
- Eliminate alcohol. Alcohol can reduce REM sleep. This is the stage of sleep when the brain and body are rejuvenated.
- If anxiety is keeping you awake, *pray.* Give all your cares and worries to God. Do this every night if necessary. Then believe HE is in control. Also, try a sleepy-time tea, valerian root capsules or calcium and magnesium. Any one of these natural substances will relax you for sleep.
- If you are a woman, it is estimated that on average, you only sleep six hours and forty minutes per night. Twenty-five percent more women suffer from insomnia than men. It is believed that hormonal ups and downs could be a contributing factor. Once hormonal levels are balanced, sleep seems to improve.

FIBER

After you complete the detoxification process, you must make sure that you continue to eliminate daily to insure that you do not become fatigued and worn out from an overaccumulation of toxins. Adding fiber to your diet will help the elimination process. Diets rich in fiber may also lower cholesterol and stabilize blood sugar levels. In addition, adding high-fiber foods to your diet will aid in the prevention and control of diabetes, colon cancer and constipation.

Oat, corn and rice bran are among the best sources of soluble fiber. Oatmeal is an excellent source of both soluble and insoluble fiber. Both quick- and long-cooking oats contain equal amounts of fiber. I like adding almonds and rice milk to my oatmeal for breakfast.

Brown rice is another wonderful choice. It has much more fiber than white rice and is more nutritious. On your eating plan be creative and cook up a large pot of brown rice; use it during the week for quick meals by adding cooked vegetables, beans and cut-up cooked chicken. Add brown rice to soups or serve it with rice milk and fruit as another breakfast choice.

Barley is also an excellent source of soluble and insoluble fiber. Add barley to soups for a satisfying meal.

Kasha, also known as buckwheat groats, has a hearty, nutlike flavor and is rich in insoluble fiber. It is wonderful as a side dish with dinner or as a stuffing for poultry.

Beans, including green peas, black-eyed peas, lentils, chickpeas and soybeans are among the best sources of soluble fiber. They are rich in protein and in minerals.

Add cooked beans to salads, casseroles and stews. Use them as a dip, or whip in a food processor and use as a sandwich spread.

Carrots, onions, broccoli and cabbage are particularly rich in soluble fiber. Broccoli and cabbage also contain substances that may have a preventive effect against some types of cancer.

Artichokes, asparagus, Brussels sprouts, celery, cauliflower, green beans, mushrooms, white and sweet potatoes with skin, alfalfa and bean and radish sprouts are good sources of insoluble fiber. Use cut-up vegetables between meals as a snack. Both baked and sweet potatoes are delicious, either alone or with leftover vegetables, herbed yogurt or melted rice cheese.

Almonds, sesame and sunflower seeds are wonderful when added to desserts, stir-frys and salads. I personally eat ten raw almonds every day. They are brimming with nutrition. Popcorn is not a major fiber source, but it is lower in fat and higher in fiber than many common snack foods.

With all of the wonderful choices you have, there should be no problem adding more fiber to your life. Substitute fiber-rich foods for foods that take away from health—like high-fat or cholesterol foods. There are also commercial fiber supplements available, such as Nature's Secret Ultimate Fiber Powder.

There is no doubt about it—fiber is good for you. By upping your fiber intake, you will not only relieve constipation but you may help prevent colon cancer as well. If you are watching your weight, you will be pleased to know that fiber will give you a feeling of fullness, which is an added bonus when you are cutting calories.

FOODS HIGH IN FIBER

- Oat bran
- Oatmeal
- Almonds
- Apple with skin
- Brown rice
- Nuts
- Seeds
- Whole-grain cereals
- Dates
- Brazil nuts
- Raisins
- Brussels sprouts (cooked)
- Papaya
- Honeydew
- Barley
- Green peas
- Lentils
- Soybeans
- Broccoli
- Artichokes
- Celery
- Green beans
- Sweet potato with skin
- Bean sprouts
- White potato with skin (baked)

- Plums
- Corn (cooked)
- Carrots (cooked)
- Pinto beans
- Raw vegetables
- Dried prunes
- Nectarine
- Pineapple
- Banana
- Spinach (cooked)
- Blueberries
- Whole cranberries
- Rice bran
- Lima beans
- Kasha
- Black-eyed peas
- Chickpeas
- Onions
- Cabbage
- Asparagus
- Cauliflower
- Mushrooms
- Alfafa
- Radish sprouts

BOWEL FUNCTION TEST

Occasionally after a detoxification program, some people experience bowel sluggishness. It is imperative that you continue to have at least two to three bowel movements per day to keep the cleansing and regeneration process moving forward smoothly. How do you accomplish this? The answer is easy enough. Just make sure that you are getting enough fiber in your diet.

A good indicator of adequate fiber intake is as follows:

· You should have a bowel movement two to three times daily.
· The stool should float.
· The stool should be almost odorless.
· The bowel movement should be effortless, no straining.
· There should be no flatulence.

Keep in mind that when you eventually eat more fiber or take a fiber supplement, you may initially experience flatulence as your body adjusts. Please make sure to drink plenty of water. This is especially true when you up your fiber intake. By making sure that your fiber intake is what it should be, you are helping to prevent dreaded ailments such as bowel cancer, colitis, constipation, diverticulitis and hemorrhoids. Just remember the stool criteria. If you see that you are off track, simply add more fiber supplements until your bowel movements are what they should be.

CALCIUM AND MAGNESIUM

Calcium, the most abundant mineral in your body, is quickly becoming a common buzz word. This wonderful mineral helps blood clotting, lowers blood pressure, prevents muscle cramping, maintains nervous system health, controls anxiety and depression and helps promote and insure a good night's sleep. Much information has been distributed about the connection between osteoporosis and the lack of calcium.

What you may not have heard is that all calcium supplementation is not created equal. Recently, I had the pleasure of doing an informative television show with chiropractor Dr. Michael Pinkus. Dr. Pinkus recommends a calcium/magnesium product that has shown dramatic results in calcium absorption. While spending time researching this formula for the television show, I began using it myself. I was amazed at the results.

Twenty-five million American women are affected by osteoporosis, which is decreased bone mass and density. Up to 50 percent of all women over the age of forty-five have or will have this dreadful disease. Five million men in this country are also affected. These are the facts. Now here is what you can do about it. Ninety-nine percent of the calcium in the body is stored in the bones and teeth. The leftover 1 percent circulates in the blood stream. This circulating calcium is needed for your heart to beat and your muscles to move. There are only two ways you can get this essential circulating calcium: first, from the calcium derived from your diet, and second, the calcium derived from your bones. By getting enough calcium from your diet, you spare your bones. Besides the structural benefits, the calcium in your bones is used to supply your blood with "emergency" doses of calcium when needed.

If that critical 1 percent of circulating calcium drops, due to calcium deficiency in your diet or because of an inferior calcium supplement, your body responds by stealing the calcium from your bones to bring the circulating calcium level back to normal. Your body has a built-in survival mechanism developed by God that knows that keeping your heart beating and your nerves firing is more important than having strong bones. The body will do anything to stay in balance, including weakening the bones to provide enough calcium for the blood. If this cycle of calcium stealing continues over time, your bones get weaker and weaker. The scary part is that you won't even feel it. Calcium deficiency does not have any real noticeable symptoms. Your first indication may be experiencing a fracture or brittle bones, especially during and after menopause.

Now we come to the most important part. I am sure that you have heard about or may even be taking a calcium supplement to protect your bones. There are even many commercials on television today about taking antacids like Tums to get your quota for calcium. Pay close attention; while Tums does contain calcium, it is an antacid. In order for calcium to be absorbed by your body, it must be in an acidic environment. Antacids dry up acid, making the calcium unabsorbable.

Dr. Pinkus showed an x-ray of a patient's abdomen with small white torpedo-shaped objects in the digestive tract. Would you believe that these objects were calcium tablets, unabsorbed and completely intact? They were going to leave the body in the same condition they were when the patient swallowed them. Not absorbed, not broken down, not effective, wouldn't you agree? Many people who take calcium supplements believe that they are doing the right thing to protect their bones, yet their bones are still brittle, their muscles are wasting, and they are weak, tired and stressed.

The reason we have this calcium-deficient epidemic occurring in the midst of the calcium supplementation craze is that very few of the supplements on the market are absorbable. The formula I tried, endorsed by Dr. Pinkus, is called CalMax Pain, Back and Stress Formula. The formula contains ascorbic acid (vitamin C) and natural lemon, which provides the slightly acidic environment that is so important for the formula to be absorbed. The formula is in powder form and dissolves in hot water; when ingested, it can be digested immediately. The calcium and magnesium in the formula absorbs through the lining in your stomach and gets into your blood quickly. This makes CalMax about ten times more absorbable than any other calcium product on the market.

We must not overlook the importance of magnesium. The next important factor in having enough calcium in the blood is magnesium. Magnesium is necessary for calcium to be absorbed into the cells. Magnesium has been linked as the critical element in over 325 biochemical reactions in the human body. Medically, magnesium is one of the most overlooked vitamins. It plays a role in hormone transmission, is responsible for muscle control and heart function (remember, the heart is a muscle) and is linked to Alzheimer's disease and learning disorders in children. According to Dr. Pinkus, any one who has had heart disease, by-pass surgery or a heart attack can benefit from taking the CalMax powder on a daily basis.

There are several substances and factors that reduce the body's levels of magnesium. They are alcohol, sugar, junk foods, pain, coffee, dieting, candida overgrowth, sodas (regular and diet), stress, surgery and diuretics. The following health conditions are associated with a magnesium deficiency: asthma, chronic fatigue syndrome, congestive heart disease, arthritis, angina, constipation, depression, fibromyalgia, ulcers, stomach problems, high cholesterol, high blood pressure, low blood sugar, insomnia, kidney stones, migraines, muscle cramps, multiple sclerosis, obesity, premenstrual syndrome, thyroid problems and stroke. So you see, magnesium is very important for optimal health as well as calcium.

As we discussed earlier in the makeover, most healing occurs at night while sleeping. If you are in pain, you can't sleep; without sleep, you cannot regenerate and heal. The result is more pain and even less sleep. The rationale behind the CalMax formula is that when taken before bed, the magnesium in the CalMax formula enters the blood stream, and within minutes, you feel your muscles relax. The calcium gets into your cells and helps repair your injured tissues. Thousands of people have reported getting a good night's sleep after drinking a cup of this formula. You sleep, your body has time to regenerate, and you feel better. It's that simple. This formula is safe for everyone—young and old, athletes, housewives, hyperactive children, executives and anyone who is trying to improve the health of their body and the quality of their calcium supplementation.

This formula is not a magic bullet. There is no such thing. Natural healing takes time. By using this highly absorbable formula of calcium and magnesium, you will give your body the best assistance in the immune-building process. CalMax works at a cellular level. It helps your body repair its own healing system on a physiological level. Remember, the very best of all possible supplementation is to supplement each day from the Word of God.

CalMax ordering information can be found at the back of this book.

CANDIDA AND CANDIDIASIS

As a child, I was given many rounds of antibiotics. As I mentioned earlier, one physician even gave me daily preventative antibiotics to prevent rheumatic fever. Antibiotics were extremely popular at that time and were given out at the hint of an illness. It was not known that the imbalance of bowel flora that antibiotics cause could lead to a systemic condition known as candidiasis. I was plagued for twenty years following constant antibiotic use with this often undiagnosed illness.

I see many unfortunate people in my practice who are from the baby-boomer generation like myself. They have a similar history of frequent antibiotic use and are suffering to the point that they feel life is no longer worth living. I too had my dark days with systemic candidiasis until I came across a wonderful book, *The Yeast Connection* by William Crook, M.D. As I read his book, I felt as though I were reading my life story. All of the case histories of people with symptoms that made the quality of life very poor were connected to a history of repeated antibiotic use. This book was a godsend to me. Because this problem of yeast involvement is present in many people with chronic complaints, I always address yeast eradication in every program of health building that I design. Yeast-related problems can affect people of all ages and affects both sexes. However, women do seem to suffer from yeast involvement more often than men. This is probably due to the rise and fall of our hormones during our monthly cycles and the way our bodies were designed. The definitive diagnosis of a yeast-connected illness is based on your health history and how your body responds to a yeast-free/sugar-free eating plan coupled with proper supplementation to address imbalances and the use of antifungal preparations.

Candida, which is a form of yeast, destroys the integrity, energy and health of the body. Candida overgrowth in the body causes an increased need for nutrients because of the pollution factor created by toxins. It has been said that this pollution factor increases your nutritional needs four to ten times above normal. If these needs are not met, then the tissues involved will break down even faster, allowing extreme conditions of sub-health and disease to exist. Large amounts of nutrients are not needed in a body that is clean, pure and healthy. This is why it is important to rid your body of this unruly guest.

Could yeast be the cause of any of your health problems? Take this candida questionnaire and score test as developed by Dr. Crook. It is designed for adults—the scoring system is not appropriate for children. It is, however, designed for both sexes. Fill out and score this questionnaire. You may be able to see the possibility of yeast overgrowth as a contributing factor to your sub-health condition, thus lowering your immune response.

Section A: History

Scoring for Section A: At the end of each question is the score for a "yes" answer.

1. Have you taken Tetracycline or other antibiotics for acne one month or longer? (35)
❑ YES   ❑ No   _____

2. Have you at any time in your life taken broad spectrum antibiotics or other antibacterial medication for respiratory, urinary or other infections for two months or longer, or in shorter courses, four or more times in a one-year period? (35)
❑ YES   ❑ No   _____

3. Have you taken a broad spectrum antibiotic drug, even in a single dose? (6)
❑ YES   ❑ No   _____

4. Have you at any time in your life been bothered by persistent prostatitis, vaginitis or other problems affecting your reproductive organs? (25)
❑ YES   ❑ No   _____

5. Are you bothered by memory or concentration problems, do you sometimes feel spaced out? (20)
❑ YES   ❑ No   _____

6. Do you feel "sick all over," yet in spite of visits to many physicians, the causes haven't been found? (20)
❑ YES   ❑ No   _____

7. Have you been pregnant:
Two or more times? (5)
❑ YES   ❑ No   _____
One time? (3)
❑ YES   ❑ No   _____

8. Have you taken birth control pills:
For more than two years? (15)
❑ YES   ❑ No   _____
For six months to two years? (8)
❑ YES   ❑ No   _____

9. Have you taken steroids orally, by injection or inhalation:
For more than two weeks? (15)
❑ YES   ❑ No   _____
For two weeks or less? (6)
❑ YES   ❑ No   _____

10. Does exposure to perfumes, insecticides, fabric shop odors and other chemicals provoke moderate to severe symptoms? (20)

❏ Yes ❏ No   _____

Mild symptoms? (5)

❏ Yes ❏ No   _____

11. Does tobacco smoke really bother you? (10)

❏ Yes ❏ No   _____

12. Are your symptoms worse on damp, muggy days or in moldy places? (20)

. ❏ Yes ❏ No   _____

13. Have you had athlete's foot, ringworm, "jock itch" or other chronic fungus infections of the skin or nails? (10)

❏ Yes ❏ No   _____

Have such infections been severe or persistent? (20)

❏ Yes ❏ No   _____

Mild to moderate? (10)

❏ Yes ❏ No   _____

14. Do you crave sugar? (10)

❏ Yes ❏ No   _____

Total Score Section A   _____

Section B: Major symptoms

These symptoms are often present in persons with yeast-connected health challenges.

Scoring system for Section B:

- Occasional or mild: 3 points.
- Frequent and/or moderately severe: 6 points.
- Severe and/or disabling: 9 points.

  1. Fatigue or lethargy   _____
  2. Feeling of being "drained"   _____
  3. Depression or manic depression   _____
  4. Numbness, burning or tingling   _____
  5. Headaches   _____
  6. Muscle aches   _____
  7. Muscle weakness or paralysis   _____
  8. Pain and/or swelling in joints   _____
  9. Abdominal pain   _____
10. Bloating, belching, or intestinal gas   _____

11. Constipation and/or diarrhea _____
12. Troublesome vaginal burning, itching, or discharge _____
13. Prostatitis _____
14. Impotence _____
15. Loss of sexual desire or feeling _____
16. Endometriosis _____
17. Cramps and/or other menstrual irregularities _____
18. Premenstrual tension _____
19. Attacks of anxiety or crying _____
20. Cold hands or feet, low body temperature _____
21. Hypothyroidism _____
22. Shaking or irritable when hungry _____
23. Cystitis or interstitial cystitis _____

Total Score Section B _____

Section C: Additional yeast-related symptoms
Scoring system for section C:
- Occasional or mild: 1 point.
- Frequent and/or moderately severe: 2 points.
- Severe and/or disabling: 3 points.

1. Drowsiness, including inappropriate drowsiness _____
2. Irritability _____
3. Incoordination _____
4. Frequent mood swings _____
5. Insomnia _____
6. Dizziness or loss of balance _____
7. Pressure above ears, feeling of head swelling _____
8. Sinus problems, tenderness of cheekbones or forehead _____
9. Tendency to bruise easily _____
10. Eczema, itching eyes _____
11. Psoriasis _____
12. Chronic hives _____
13. Indigestion or heartburn _____
14. Sensitivity to milk, wheat, corn or other common foods _____
15. Mucus in stools _____
16. Rectal itching _____

17. Dry mouth or throat   _____
18. Mouth rashes, including "white tongue"   _____
19. Bad breath   _____
20. Foot, hair or body odor not relieved by washing   _____
21. Nasal congestion or postnasal drip   _____
22. Nasal itching   _____
23. Sore throat   _____
24. Laryngitis, loss of voice   _____
25. Cough or recurrent bronchitis   _____
26. Pain or tightness in chest   _____
27. Wheezing or shortness of breath   _____
28. Urinary frequency or urgency   _____
29. Burning on urination   _____
30. Spots in front of eyes or erratic vision   _____
31. Burning or tearing eyes   _____
32. Recurrent infections or fluid in ears   _____
33. Ear pain or deafness   _____

Total Score Section C   _____

Total Score
                              Section A   _____
                              Section B   _____
                              Section C   _____

GRAND TOTAL SCORE   _____

How did you score? Women with a score over 180 and men with a score over 140 almost certainly have yeast-connected health problems. Women with a score over 120 and men with a score over 90 probably have yeast-connected health problems. Yeast-connected health problems are possibly present in women with scores over 60 and in men with scores over 40. With scores less than 60 in women and less than 40 in men, yeasts are less apt to be the cause of your health problems.

Most of the people that I have worked with in my office have scored very high on the yeast questionnaire. And most of these people are the product of the antibiotic era. As you can see, there are a number of possible symptoms that yeast overgrowth can cause in your body. Many people, including myself, had a physician for virtually every system of their body. In his classic book on yeast, *The Missing Diagnosis*, Dr. C. Orian Truss said:

> Each woman with this problem will have experienced during the course of the illness perhaps 80 percent or more of the many manifestations that characterize this chronic yeast problem. This condition is devastating to a woman's ability to function, whether in a career, as a wife and mother, or outside the home. Its unpredictability often makes it impossible to plan activities requiring more than minimal responsibility.

This is exactly what happened to me as a result of yeast involvement. Once I learned the cause—which, by the way, took years to discover—thanks to the work of Dr. Crook and Dr. Truss, I was armed with the knowledge and wisdom to begin my journey back to health. Dr. Truss continued to say in *The Missing Diagnosis*, "Women with this condition can show great fortitude, and can accept the fact that patience and time will be required for a full recovery."

Rest in the LORD and wait patiently for Him.

— PSALM 37:7, NKJV

During this phase, we will continue the same eating plan as in the first 30 days. Notice that it is free of yeast, dairy products and sugar. This is the optimal way to eat, not only for immune health building, but for yeast eradication also. It has proven itself time and time again because of its twofold effect. It builds health while discouraging and suppressing further yeast overgrowth. If you scored high or relatively high on the yeast questionnaire, you need to implement the following supplements and lifestyle changes during this 60-day phase. You will continue with the 30-day supplements and simply add the following to the program (you may choose any of the following protocols for yeast eradication):

- For a high score: Candistroy by Nature's Secret, developed by Lindsey Duncan. Follow the directions on the box.

- For a moderate score: Kyolic Garlic Liquid is antifungal; acidophilus liquid restocks the intestinal pond; caprylic acid is antifungal; grapefruit seed extract is antifungal. Kyolic is incredibly effective by itself along with acidophilus. Pick only one antifungal at a time because of the potential die-off reactions, which will be explained later.

- For a low score: Pau de Arco tea is antifungal. Start slow—this is powerful. Begin with ½ cup twice weekly; sweeten with stevia extract. Also, incorporate garlic into your cooking or take Kyolic Garlic capsules or liquid daily.

WHAT CAN YOU EAT?

Here are several great recipes that build your immunity and promote regeneration while discouraging further yeast overgrowth. These dishes are to be incorporated in your immune-boosting eating plan. Enjoy!

CABBAGE SOUP

1 medium head of cabbage, cut into 2-in. pieces (9 c.)
2 large onions, diced (2 c.)
4 cloves garlic, thinly sliced
3¼ c. water
1 can (28 oz.) crushed tomatoes
1 tsp. oregano
1 clove

Place cabbage, onion, garlic and 1 cup water in a Dutch oven set over moderate heat. Cook until cabbage has wilted, about 10 minutes. Add remaining water, tomatoes, oregano and clove. After bringing to a boil, reduce to a simmer. Cook for 45 minutes. Serves 4.

HEALTHY VEGETABLE CHILI

¼ c. olive oil
2 medium onions, diced in ½-in. pieces
2 large sweet red peppers, diced in ¼-in. pieces
4 cloves garlic, minced
2 medium zucchini, diced in ½-in. pieces
1 can (35 oz.) Italian plum tomatoes, chopped
1½ lb. ripe plum tomatoes, diced in 1-in. pieces
½ c. chopped fresh parsley
2 Tbsp. chili powder (not hot)
1 Tbsp. each dried basil, oregano and ground cumin
1 tsp. each fennel seed and pepper
1 c. each cooked kidney and garbanzo beans
½ c. chopped fresh dill
2 Tbsp. lemon juice

Cook onion, pepper and garlic in 2 tablespoons of oil in a Dutch oven over low heat until soft, about 7 minutes. Add remaining oil and zucchini; stir to coat. Add tomatoes, parsley and spices; simmer 30 minutes. Stir in kidney beans, garbanzo beans, dill and lemon juice. Simmer 15 minutes. Serves 4.

GREEK MILLET SANDWICH

Nonstick spray
¼ c. chopped onion
¼ c. green pepper
2 cloves garlic, minced
1 boned and skinned chicken breast, halved and cut into ½-in. cubes
¼ c. diced sun-dried tomatoes
3 pitted olives, sliced
¼ tsp. dried basil, crumbled
¼ c. rice cheese (you may add a small amount of feta)
2 medium-size millet flats, warmed and split open to form a pocket

Spray a medium-size skillet with nonstick spray and set over moderate heat. Add onion, pepper and garlic and cook, stirring occasionally until onion has softened, about 5 minutes. Add chicken and cook until no longer pink, 4 to 5 minutes. Add tomatoes, olives and basil; cook 1 minute. Remove from heat, stir in cheese and spoon into warmed millet bread pocket. Serves 2.

RATATOUILLE

2 Tbsp. olive oil
1 large onion, halved and thinly sliced (1 c.)
3 cloves garlic, minced
3 medium zucchini, thinly sliced
1 large red, yellow or green pepper (or a combo of all), diced
1 medium eggplant, cubed
5 medium tomatoes, chopped
1 bay leaf
½ tsp. dried marjoram
1 tsp. each dried basil and oregano, crumbled
½ c. plain toasted millet bread crumbs

Heat oil in a Dutch oven set over moderate heat. Add onion and garlic; cook, stirring occasionally until softened, about 7 minutes. Add zucchini, pepper and eggplant; cover and cook 10 minutes, stirring occasionally. Add tomatoes, bay leaf, dried marjoram, basil and oregano; cook uncovered, stirring occasionally until vegetables are tender and dish has thickened, about 15 to 20 minutes. Remove bay leaf. Add bread crumbs if you would like a thicker comfort food. Serves 4.

FOODS YOU CAN EAT FREELY

- All fresh vegetables (except carrots and beets) and vegetable juices
- All fish (except scavengers and shellfish). Deep-sea white fish and salmon are particularly good.
- Stevia as a sweetener
- Free-range meats, ideally chicken and turkey
- Eggs
- Purified water
- Lemons, limes, cranberries and Granny Smith apples
- Grapefruit and kiwi (after 20–60 days)
- Well-cooked grains: millet, buckwheat, amaranth, quinoa–NO WHEAT!
- Pasta made from the above grains
- Essential fatty acids (Ultimate Oil and olive oil)
- Beans, grits, raw almonds and seeds
- Pau de Arco tea

FOODS TO AVOID

- Sugars: sucrose, fructose, maltose, lactose, glucose, mannitol, sorbitol, maple syrup, sugar, brown sugar, raw sugar, date sugar, corn syrup and honey
- Aspartame and NutraSweet
- Yeast-containing foods, breads and pastries
- Alcohol, soda, coffee and fermented beverages (like cider)
- Cheese and sour milk products (sour cream and buttermilk)
- All nuts (except raw almonds)
- Mayonnaise, mustard and ketchup
- Fruit (except ones mentioned above)
- Mushrooms (remember, yeast is a fungus)

SIXTY DAYS "DIE-OFF" (HERXHEIMER REACTION)

Die-off is the natural process that occurs when you kill colonies of yeast throughout your body. If you are following the yeast-free, dairy-free, sugar-free eating plan and are taking antifungal supplements like Candistroy, Kyolic Garlic, caprylic acid, grapefruit seed extract or Pau de Arco tea, you are bound to experience this often misunderstood phenomenon. Here's what occurs. On an effective program, thousands upon thousands of yeast cells are dying very quickly. Yeast poisons or toxins are being created faster than the immune system or eliminative channels can remove from the blood. Therefore, you may feel some of the temporary discomforts such as headache, fatigue, muscle aches, joint or chest pain, sinus, lung, throat inflammation and mucus, congestion, gas, dizziness, mild depression and others.

These symptoms are usually short lived if you are following your plan correctly. However, there are times when a rest from the antifungals is recommended while continuing to eat yeast, sugar and dairy free. A rest of ten days from the antifungals will calm any harsh die-off symptoms, or you may discontinue the antifungals after 60 days. You may need to take them periodically to keep the yeast in check.

Persons not familiar with the die-off reaction feel as though this process is something detrimental to their health. They are so conditioned to feeling bad that it has become a way of life for them to focus on the negative instead of the very positive process occurring within their bodies. I have experienced the die-off reaction

104

many times. The best way to describe it is that it resembles the flu. The severity of the symptoms seems to depend upon the amount of yeast being killed and your body's ability to eliminate the yeast. If you are feeling flulike and achy, that's wonderful! The program is working! Stay with it and follow through. The only way to overcome yeast overgrowth is to starve it, kill it and then remove it from your system.

Again, if the symptoms are especially uncomfortable, simply take one to ten days off from the antifungals, drink plenty of water with lemon and take the salt-and-soda detoxifying bath mentioned in the first 30-days section. Press forward toward the prize. It is a journey that will leave you amazed. You will become very well acquainted with your body, probably for the first time in your life. You will become more aware of how important it is to take special care of your body so that you will not have to experience dieoff and all of its uncomfortable symptoms. Relax! God is in charge.

ENZYMES— IMPROVED IMMUNE FUNCTION

Enzymes are crucial. They turn the foods that we eat into energy and unlock this energy for use in the body. Enzymes have far-reaching benefits. They deliver nutrients, carry away toxic wastes, digest food, purify the blood, deliver hormones by feeding and fortifying the endocrine system, balance cholesterol and triglyceride levels, feed the brain and cause no harm to the body. The strength of our enzyme activity is important in building a stronger immune system as well as healthier blood. Our bodies make two basic types of enzymes: digestive and metabolic. Our bodies secrete digestive enzymes to help us break down food into nutrients and wastes. Our digestive enzymes include pepsin, lipase, protease, amylase, trypsin and ptyalin. Metabolic enzymes speed up the chemical reaction within the cells for detoxification and energy production. These enzymes enable us to see, hear, feel, move and think. Every organ, every tissue and all 100 trillion cells in our body depend upon the reaction of metabolic enzymes and their energy factor. Metabolic enzymes are produced by the liver, pancreas, gallbladder and other organs.

We also receive enzymes from raw foods that we eat and by taking enzyme supplements. I strongly recommend that you supplement your body with enzymes. Why? The answer is plain common sense. In our busy lifestyles and hectic schedules, we overcook, microwave and overprocess our foods—killing all or most of the enzymes. While it's true that we occasionally eat raw foods that contain live enzyme activity, our consumption of cooked "dead enzyme" foods is greater. This leaves our bodies a big job of producing more enzymes to break down these cooked foods unless we supplement. I have seen people gain more energy, lose weight, sleep better and feel better in general after supplementing their bodies with enzymes. This is because our bodies work more efficiently with proper enzyme activity. No excess energy has to be expended by the body on the process of digestion. It has been said that we are only as healthy as what we assimilate and eliminate. At this 60-day mark, you will assimilate or digest better with the help of supplemental enzymes and eliminate better by detoxifying your body.

A variety of supplemental enzymes are available through different sources. It is very important that you use an enzyme supplement tailored to your particular situation. Also, you must make sure that the doses are measured in active units, which are the most potent. In my research, I have found that there are four basic types of enzyme deficiencies. A lack of protease limits your ability to digest proteins. A lack of lipase hampers your ability to digest fats. A deficiency of amylase affects your ability to digest carbohydrates. A deficiency of any two or all three enzymes can lower the quality of your life because of lowered immune response. Additional benefits to therapeutic enzyme therapy are numerous. If we fortify the endocrine system, get the bowels working regularly and digest our food with the help of enzymes instead of turning it to fat, then we can be truly successful at losing weight and gaining energy.

Younger-looking skin is an additional benefit of proper enzyme supplementation. Enzymes can fight the aging process by increasing the blood supply to the skin, delivering life-giving nutrients and then carrying away waste products that can make your skin look old, tired and wrinkled. Because circulation slows down as we age, enzyme supplementation becomes crucial as we grow older.

Now, what type of enzymes do you take? When it comes to supplemental enzymes there are two sources: plant and animal. Personally, I use plant enzymes, as do my clients, simply because animal enzymes, commonly known as pancreatic enzymes, come from the pancreas of slaughterhouse animals. Ask yourself, Am I going to risk supplementing my body with enzymes taken from the pancreas of an animal that may have been in poor health and had cancer or any other disease? In addition, animal enzymes are not as digestively active as plant enzymes. Plant enzymes are superior and work throughout the entire digestive system and in the blood. They become active as soon as they enter the body. Not all enzyme products are alike or equal in their activity in the body. Look for the appropriate codes approved by the FDA to insure active enzyme activity. Also watch for fillers such as leftover fibers and cellulose added to the formula. Look for an enzyme supplier that uses a standard system for ensuring the potency of their enzymes. The system for determining enzyme potency used by the American Food Industry is derived from the Food and Chemical Code, or FCC. Find an enzyme supplier that measures and reports the enzyme product levels in FCC units. This way you will be assured of active, potent enzyme activity. I have found a wonderful company by the name of Enzymedica, located in Punta Gorda, Florida, that manufactures a superior line of enzymes I use exclusively in my practice. They meet all of the criteria for activity and potency. Furthermore, they have formulas specifically tailored to the four deficiency syndromes. The first formula is called Digest. This formula speeds digestion of food while reducing the body's need to produce digestive enzymes. Take one capsule with each meal. One capsule is usually sufficient for alleviating poor digestion. If you are in poor health, you may need two to five capsules until your digestion improves. Digest contains high-potency multiple enzymes along with lactobacillus acidophilus to help maintain healthy bowel flora. This formula helps you to digest protein, starch, fat, sugar and fiber.

The next formula is Purify. It contains the highest available potency of protease to help digest protein invaders in the blood. This would include parasites, fungi, bacteria and viruses that are covered by a protein film. The enzyme protease breaks down the undigested protein, toxins and debris in the blood, thereby unburdening the immune system so it can concentrate its full action. The recommended dosage is three capsules first thing in the morning and right before bed. This formula is excellent for candida sufferers who traditionally have difficulty with protein digestion and tend to have a toxic load in their bloodstream.

The next formula is Lypo. This is an excellent formula containing the highest available potency of lipase, which digests fats in the blood and digestive tract. This will help to lower cholesterol and triglycerides. It provides additional support for carbohydrates and dairy products, and it aids elimination. The recommended dosage is two capsules with each meal. If you are overweight, meaning more than twelve pounds over your ideal weight, the dosage is three capsules with meals. Usually, people who are obese are low in lipase according to research.

Gastro is the last formula on the list of these super-enzymes. This formula helps to soothe the gastrointestinal system and alleviate abdominal discomfort. It also helps relieve the burning and irritation that some people experience with digestion.

You can see that enzymes can greatly improve your life. I call them *God's sparks of life*. Look at the following chart to determine which enzymes you are deficient in.

AMYLASE DEFICIENCY

- Breaking out of skin rashes
- Depression
- Allergies
- Hot flashes
- Cold hands and feet
- Sprue
- Hypoglycemia
- Mood swings
- PMS
- Fatigue
- Neck and shoulder aches
- Inflammation

PROTEASE DEFICIENCY

- Back weakness
- Constipation
- Insomnia
- Parasites
- Gingivitis
- Fungal forms
- High blood pressure
- Hearing problems
- Gum disorders

LIPASE DEFICIENCY

- Aching feet, arthritis
- Cystitis
- Gallbladder stress
- Hay fever
- Psoriasis
- Constipation
- Heart problems
- Bladder problems
- Acne
- Gallstones
- Prostate problems
- Urinary weakness
- Diarrhea

COMBINATION DEFICIENCY

- Chronic allergies
- Diverticulitis
- Chronic fatigue
- Immune-depressed conditions
- Common colds
- Irritable bowel
- Sinus infection

By beginning your enzyme supplementation during this phase of the 90-Day Immune System Makeover, we will help the body complete the digestive process without overstressing the body's enzyme-making potential. We will then be in a much more favorable position to fight biological and system malfunctions while boosting our immune system to a higher level.

Plant enzymes help to develop and maintain a proper digestive system and can be used in varying formulas to treat certain ailments. How and when should you take your oral plant enzymes? In order for the plant enzymes to provide all the benefits during the digestion process, they need to be taken when their activity will be compatible with what is occurring during digestion. I instruct my clients to take their enzymes at the beginning of the meal because they have higher effectiveness in digesting food. Enzymes could be taken at the end of the meal, but the rate of efficiency will not be as good due to the fact that acidity has been built up during the digestive process, thereby lessening some of the enzymes' effects that have low pH. According to "The White Paper" by Dr. M. Mamadou, microbiologist and enzymologist, "for complete assimilation it is recommended that oral enzymes be taken at the beginning of the meal, halfway during the meal and at the end of the meal. If not, you may just take them at the beginning of the meal."

Once you determine your particular enzyme deficiency, you may then choose the Enzymedica plant enzyme formula that bests suits your profile.

1. **Gastro** contains amylase, lipase, cellulose, marshmallow root, gotu kola, papaya leaf and prickly ash bark. Gastro helps to alleviate conditions associated with gastro-intestinal distress, such as gout, heartburn, colitis, hiatal hernia, Crohn's disease, gastritis, unexplained blood in the urine and diverticulosis. It has a soothing effect on inflamed mucous membranes of the respiratory and gastrointestinal tract. If you suffer from gout, marshmallow root helps eliminate uric acid from the body. The recommended dosage is two to four capsules with every meal or snack.

2. **Lypo** was formulated with more lipase than the other formulas. This will help you if you suffer from heart problems, high blood pressure, plaque buildup in the arteries and obesity. For the reduction of cholesterol, it is recommended that you take two or more capsules with each meal. Lypo improves fat digestion, helps fat reduction, lowers triglycerides and balances fatty acids. For obesity, the dosage is three capsules with meals.

3. **Purify** is indicated for protease deficiency with the following indications: hypoglycemia, hepatitis, fungal infections, parasites, kidney problems, abscesses, virus infections, osteoporosis, anxiety syndromes and inflammatory conditions of the throat, nose, mouth, ear, sinus and gums. It is an all-natural blood enhancer. The recommended dosage is three capsules on an empty stomach first thing in the morning and just before bed.

4. **Digest** is indicated if you fit the following profile: dairy intolerance, sugar intolerance, food allergies, gallbladder stress, indigestion and most digestive disorders. The recommended dosage is one to five capsules with every meal and one to two capsules with snacks.

Ordering information is located at the back of the book.

In her informative book *The Healing Power of Enzymes,* DicQie Fuller, Ph.D., D.Sc., answers common questions about enzyme supplementation and provides case histories of people whose health has been restored by the use of the right enzymes. She says, "Anytime we suffer from an acute or chronic illness it is almost certain an enzyme depletion exists." She discusses candida and recommends 600,000 units of protease, three to five times a day, to help digest the spores of the fungal form of candida. She also agrees that sugar must go. She feels that it is "far easier to give up the sweets and start to rebuild our system, rather than suffer the aches, pains and swelling that come with a sugar habit." In addition, she has found that large doses of amylase help to eliminate swelling and inflammation in the body almost immediately. I highly recommend that you add her book to your library if you want to learn more about enzymes.

Enzymes and fibromyalgia

In the 90-Day Immune System Makeover, we are going to the root of chronic sub-health conditions. Take fibromyalgia, for example. I have found by applying the principles you have learned thus far—rest, therapeutic enzymes and a yeast-, sugar-, and dairy-free diet—have relieved even the most severe cases of this chronic invisible illness. My point once again: It does not matter what label your condition has. It is only that—a label. We must eliminate the toxins, yeasts and unhealthy lifestyles that contributed to current disease and regenerate your body at the cellular level.

PROBIOTICS—
GASTROINTESTINAL DEFENDERS

If you are battling any kind of digestive or intestinal problem, probiotics are a must. These gastrointestinal defenders are crucial in keeping your immune defenses in good working order. These defenders known as probiotics consist mainly of lactobacillus acidophilus and lactobacillus bifidus. They produce volatile fatty acids that provide metabolic energy. In addition, they help you digest food and amino acids, produce certain vitamins and most importantly make your lower intestine mildly acidic, which inhibits the growth of bad bacteria such as *E. coli,* which has caused serious illnesses in recent years.

Probiotic supplementation is absolutely essential in your fight against candida or any fungal infection because of the antifungal properties that these defenders possess. According to Dr. James F. Balch in his best-selling book entitled *Prescription for Nutritional Healing,* the flora in a healthy colon should consist of at least 85 percent lactobacilli and 15 percent coliform bacteria. The typical colon bacteria count today is the reverse, which has resulted in gas, bloating, intestinal and systemic toxicity, constipation and malabsorption of nutrients, making it a perfect environment for the overgrowth of candida. By adding probiotics—that is, lactobacillus acidophillus and lactobacillus bididus supplements to your system—you will return your intestinal flora to a healthier balance and eliminate all of the problems of intestinal flora imbalance mentioned.

If you are on antibiotic therapy, it is vitally important that you supplement your digestive tract with probiotics, or "good bacteria," because antibiotic use destroys your healthy bowel flora along with the harmful bacteria. Both *L. acidophilus* and *L. bifidus* promote proper digestion, help to normalize bowel function and prevent gas and candida overgrowth. This in turn keeps immunity high.

Store your probiotic formula in a cool dry place. Some brands require refrigeration. I personally prefer and use Kyo-Dophilus from Wakunaga of America because it is milk free and remains viable and stable, even at high temperatures. It contains 1.5 billion live cells per capsule, is suitable for all ages and contains *L. acidophilus, B. bifidum* and *B. longum* in a vegetable starch complex. In addition, it is free of preservatives, sugar, sodium, yeast, gluten, artificial colors and flavors and, as mentioned before, milk.

As a dietary supplement, take one capsule with a meal twice daily. Children under four should take ½ capsule with a meal twice daily. If the child cannot swallow the capsule, simply open it and sprinkle in juice or on food.

FOCUS ON FATS

That's right. Focus on fats. By this, I mean the right kind of fats. I'm talking about fatty acids that are so necessary for good health that they are called essential fatty acids. At this point in your makeover, we will add essential fatty acids, which will in turn have a positive effect on many areas of your system. Since we are focusing on candida eradication at this 60-day section, you should know that essential fatty acids are beneficial in the candida removal and system regeneration process. Essential fatty acids, commonly known as EFAs help to improve the texture and condition of your skin and hair. They aid in arthritis prevention and treatment. They help to lower cholesterol and triglyceride levels. They also help lower blood pressure, help alleviate psoriasis and eczema and are crucial in nerve impulse transmission in the brain, thereby improving brain function. EFAs are used by our bodies in the production of prostaglandins, which act as regulators and messengers of certain body processes.

How important are EFAs? All living cells need essential fatty acids. There are two main types of EFAs. The first is called Omega 3, which can be found in deep-water fish like salmon, mackerel and sardines, canola oil and my favorite, flaxseed oil. The second type of EFA is called Omega 6, which an be found in grape seed oil, sesame oil, vegetable oil, soybean oil, seeds, nuts and legumes.

When it comes to supplementation, there are several ways to go. First, you may add any of the above-mentioned food sources to your eating plan to insure adequate EFA intake, or you may supplement with the following supplements that I have found to be very good in clinical use.

For Omega 3:

- Flaxseed oil, capsules or liquid, can aid arthritis relief and lower cholesterol and triglyceride levels.
- Carlson Salmon Oil, liquid or capsules, is excellent for arthritis.

Combination Omega 3 and Omega 6:

- Nature's Secret Ultimate Oil: Follow directions on label.

- Wakunaga's Kyolic EPA—follow manufacturers directions on dosage.

These are my personal favorites, because you get the best of both worlds—Omega 3 and Omega 6 fatty acids. You should add whichever you choose to your program at this 60-day point. In addition, as you prepare your meals, use only olive oil in your food preparation. Olive oil reduces the amount of LDL in the bloodstream. It has been said that incorporating olive oil in your diet can lower your LDL levels better than eating a low-fat diet. In order for cholesterol levels to drop, however, you must add fiber in addition to olive oil and your EFA combination Omega 3 and Omega 6 formula.

Please note that even though you will find most of your natural oils in dark containers to keep out light, keep them in the refrigerator and use them quickly because they can go rancid. If you cannot use a bottle of oil in a month, then purchase a smaller bottle. This is especially true if you choose flaxseed oil. I keep my combination Nature's Secret Ultimate Oil or Kyolic-EPA in my refrigerator even though it is not imperative that you do so.

Natural Antibiotics

Right now, you may be asking yourself, If antibiotics can contribute to yeast overgrowth, what can I use to treat any infection that may arise after I have gone through the yeast eradication program? You will be pleased to know that there are many natural substances that are powerful antibiotics to choose from. The first one is biotic silver, a pure silver protein. It is a very powerful natural antibiotic and antifungal solution that is so strong and effective that it kills and removes from the body all bacteria, viruses and fungi within a short period of time. According to Gary Carlson, director of the Candida Wellness Center in Provo, Utah, this natural antibiotic is extremely effective and overcomes serious infections. It has been approved by the Federal Drug Administration and is classified as a "Dietary Mineral Supplement." There are no side effects recorded in decades of use, and studies at the University of Toronto concluded that no toxicity, even in high dosages, results from using biotic silver.

Having sufficient pure silver protein in the body is like having a superior second immune system. Long ago, when the earth was more fertile and our food supply was more pure and natural, there was more silver in the soil, and it would be absorbed into our food. In minute amounts, this silver would prevent infectious disease because no yeast, bacteria or virus can survive in the presence of silver. But today, due to the mining of silver for its monetary value and the inorganic methods of farming, there is little silver left in the soil. In addition, strains of infectious organisms are so much stronger today that larger than normal amounts of silver are necessary to eradicate them.

Research indicates that biotic silver protein has been used successfully in the treatment of more than 650 diseases, including allergies, athlete's foot, pneumonia, pleurisy, bladder infections, boils, candida yeast infections, cold sores, cold, flu, cystitis, dermatitis, fungal infection, indigestion, lupus, lyme disease, malaria, psoriasis, rhinitis, ringworm, sinus infections, staph, tonsillitis, viruses of all forms, warts and whooping cough. Biotic silver has been found to be both a remedy and prevention for all colds, flu, infections, bacteria, fungi and viruses, including staph and strep.

I know you are probably excited about this wonderful product. However, you must know the difference between colloidal silver and biotic silver. Biotic silver is the most advanced form of colloidal silver for the therapeutic purpose of fighting infection available today. The superior effect comes from a special scientific process that allows it to reach negative microorganisms quickly and destroy them completely everywhere in the body. Once the pure silver protein has accomplished its goal, it is removed from the body with no toxic accumulation or side effects.

Silver particle size is important when it comes to a superior silver protein formula. In the case of biotic silver, it is certified to have silver particles down to .001 microns or smaller, which allows the particles to flow freely through even the smallest capillaries of the body and enter and be removed completely from the cells and tissues. It is a product that is well designed and formulated from the finest research and scientific achievements in the fields of parasitology and probiotics. It can even be given to infants and be used during pregnancy. Because it is a special proprietary formulation, it does no harm to human enzymes, hormones or any part of the body chemistry. Tests in hospitals, universities and research laboratories have proven this beyond a doubt. No one has ever overdosed, and it is not an allopathic poison. It is goldish in color, tasteless, odorless and does not upset the stomach. It is nontoxic, nonaddictive, nonaccumulative and completely safe.

For ordering information, see the references and product source section at the back of the book.

Other choices of natural antibiotics include goldenseal, grapefruit seed concentrate, oil of oregano and olive leaf extract. These can be found in your local health food store. Olive leaf is a 100 percent natural, herbal antibacterial, antiviral and antifungal extract taken from specific parts of the olive tree. In addition, it is a nontoxic immune system builder. Recently a more concentrated form of olive leaf extract has been developed and is marketed under the name of Defend. Several long-term sufferers of chronic fungal infections have noticed regression or clearing faster than any previously used product. According to Gary Carlson, many individuals with fibromyalgia, Epstein-Barr virus, long-term infections and chronic fatigue syndrome are reporting feeling much better with more complete relief when taking Defend. Olive leaf may also be a potent tool against the common cold and flu. Other benefits that researchers have found is that olive leaf could lower blood sugar, rid people of bladder infections, asthma, swollen glands, scalp and skin conditions, sinus infections and more.

Goldenseal acts as an antibiotic and has anti-inflammatory and antibacterial properties. It is good for any infectious disease. If you use it at the first sign of cold, flu or sore throat, it may stop it from developing further. If it doesn't stop it, it will shorten the duration of the symptoms. Oil of oregano is a very powerful antibacterial agent. Use it very sparingly. Grapefruit seed extract is antifungal, antibacterial, and antiviral. It is available in a liquid or capsule form. Nasal sprays are also available.

THYROID HEALTH AND THE IMMUNE SYSTEM

Your thyroid gland is the thermostat of your body. It produces hormones to help keep your metabolic rate stable and to keep energy-producing and energy-using processes in balance. If it is depleted or deficient, the rest of the body functions improperly, which leads to lower immunity. Thyroid problems can cause many recurring illnesses and fatigue. To test yourself for an underactive thyroid, take this self-test developed by Broda Barnes, M.D., author of *Hypothyroidism: The Unsuspected Illness.* This test is well known in the field of natural medicine and is used routinely.

Keep a basal thermometer by your bedside. Before turning in, shake down the thermometer and place it within easy reach of your bed. In the morning, before arising, lie still, and place it under your armpit for ten minutes. Keep quiet and still—any motion can upset the reading. This is done for seven to ten days consecutively. Women should not take a reading during the first few days of their menstrual cycle or on the middle day of their cycle because body temperature fluctuates during those times. A normal reading is between 97.8 and 98.2. A temperature below 97.6 degrees Fahrenheit may indicate low thyroid function. Record your readings for the next ten days in the following spaces.

DATE   TEMPERATURE

1. _____   _____

2. _____   _____

3. _____   _____

4. _____   _____

5. _____   _____

6. _____   _____

7. _____   _____

8. _____   _____

9. _____   _____

10. _____   _____

If your temperature is consistently below 97.6, you should add the following supplements to your 90-Day Immune System Makeover program, or see your physician for Armor Thyroid, which is available by prescription only.

- Kelp—contains iodine
- Raw thyroid glandular—helps to replace deficient thyroid hormone
- B-complex vitamin—helps improve thyroid function and immune function
- Essential fatty acids—necessary for proper thyroid gland function

ADRENAL GLANDS— YOUR BODY'S BATTERIES

One of the most important areas to rebuild when it comes to stronger immunity is your glandular system. Of particular importance are the two little glands that sit on top of each kidney known as the adrenal glands.

The adrenal glands help your body deal with stress. They secrete adrenaline in crisis situations to give you extra energy to handle an immediate crisis. Built into our wonderfully designed bodies is a response to immediate danger known as the "fight or flight" response. Years ago when our society was not so stress laden, this came in handy when a dangerous situation arose, whether it was during battle or running from a lion or tiger. The trouble today is that many of us have fallen victim to chronic, unremitting stress. Our adrenal glands are producing an almost constant stream of adrenaline, causing us to feel stressed out, hyped up and finally, fatigued. These glands are depleted and taxed by all of this stress, compounded with excessive caffeine and sugar consumption, lack of sleep and poor diet. When your adrenal glands are zapped by all of the above, your immune system suffers, and you can fall victim to stress-related illness, including allergies.

The adrenal glands are made up of two parts: the cortex, which is responsible for cortisone production, and the medulla, which secretes the adrenaline. The adrenal cortex helps to maintain body balance, regulates sugar and carbohydrates, metabolism and produces sex hormones. The adrenal medulla produces epinephrine or adrenaline and norepinephrine to speed up the metabolism in times of stress. Long-term use of corticosteroids can impair adrenal function and cause them to shrink in size.

Some of the symptoms of adrenal gland exhaustion or fatigue are lack of energy, feeling anxious, weakness, lethargy, poor memory, moodiness and irritability, hypoglycemia, diabetes, low immunity, dry skin, brittle nails and food cravings, especially for sugar. As you can see, the adrenal glands are crucial to optimal immunity. A good diet is essential for proper adrenal health. The eating plan on the 90-Day Immune System Makeover is perfect for adrenal health, because it is low in sugar and fats. In addition, it contains brown rice and seafood, which are adrenal-building foods.

Exercise aids in adrenal health because it helps you release tension and stress. Sleep is also crucial when it comes to recharging your adrenal glands. As a matter of fact, sleep recharges your entire body, so make proper rest a habit.

If you feel that your adrenal glands need recharging, you should supplement your body with the following:

- Pantothenic acid, 500–2000 mg. daily
- B-complex vitamins
- Vitamin C, 3,000 mg. daily
- Royal jelly, 2 tsp. daily
- Astragalus, as directed
- An adrenal complex glandular

An adrenal complex glandular will help nourish and stimulate your exhausted adrenals. It helps to reduce inflammation and increases body tone and endurance. It helps protect against chronic fatigue syndrome and candida albicans, as well as helping to overcome allergies. It works with vitamin B and vitamin C to overcome blood sugar imbalances, as in hypoglycemia and diabetes.

Adrenal gland function test

If you want to see how well your adrenal glands are performing, try this self-test. Get yourself a blood pressure home test kit. First lie down and rest for about five minutes. Then take your blood pressure. Stand up immediately and take your blood pressure reading again. If your blood pressure is lower after you stand up, you probably have reduced adrenal gland performance. The lower it is from your resting blood pressure reading, the more severe the low adrenal function. The systolic number (or the number on top of the blood pressure reading) normally is about ten points higher when you are standing than when you lie down. If you see a difference of more than ten points, you should address adrenal health right away as this will only enhance your immune health and well-being.

HORMONES AND HEALTH

Is this section just for women? Most definitely not! Men have hormones, too. There seems to be an epidemic of hormone-related cancers in the past forty years. This is something we need to explore further. Let me share with you some very important information that may shock you at first, but will arm you with the knowledge you need to prevent hormonal imbalance that appears to be behind this upswing in cancers that are hormonally driven.

If you are a woman and are considering using hormone replacement therapy, that is, estrogen or estrogen and progestin, it's imperative to learn how to make an informed choice. The choice you make can and will have a tremendous impact on your current and future health. Because this book is not about hormonal imbalance, I highly recommend that you read *What Your Doctor May Not Tell You About Menopause* by Dr. John R. Lee. I had the pleasure of meeting Dr. Lee in 1998 while filming a television show in Orlando. I had studied Dr. Lee's work concerning the importance of natural progesterone as estrogen's natural balancer. I can personally attest to this as I have battled hormonal imbalance for the past twenty years. Natural progesterone cream has balanced my system in addition to the immune makeover lifestyle changes.

Our environment these days contains estrogen mimics known as xenobiotics. Xenobiotics have a profound impact on hormone balance. Most xenobiotics are petrochemically based. Because of the widespread use of petrochemicals, they are difficult to avoid. Here is a list of some products that are currently made from petrochemicals or actually contain them: perfumes, pesticides, soaps, clothing, medicines, microchips, plastics and many more. I won't argue that these substances have greatly improved our quality of life, but we are paying a price. We are polluting our bodies, air, water and soil with these petrochemicals. Because of their estrogenic effect, there is an epidemic of reproductive abnormalities, which include increasing numbers of cancers of the reproductive systems in both men and women, infertility and low sperm counts. Estrogenic effect simply means having an estrogen-like effect upon the body. This effect can promote cell division in the breast and uterine lining. In men it can contribute to hormonal imbalance that can play a part in reproductive health issues.

According to Dr. Lee, the potential consequences of this overexposure are staggering, especially considering that one of the consequences is passing on reproductive abnormalities to offspring. These xenobiotics are commonly referred to as xenoestrogens because of their estrogenic effects on both male and female physiology.

The good news is that we can reduce our exposure to these potentially dangerous chemical estrogen mimics.

You can protect your children and grandchildren by doing the following:

· Refuse to use pesticides.
· Limit use of plastics.
· Drink out of glass containers instead of plastic.
· Purchase hormone-free meat and organic produce.
· Use natural green products for detergents and household cleaners.
· Use natural products instead of petrochemical products.

This may cost more, but not as much as losing your health. In addition, if you are a woman who is experiencing PMS, premenopause or menopausal symptoms, the use of natural progesterone as a balancer for dominant estrogen levels has been a godsend for many ailing women. Most of the symptoms that women experience, such as migraines, bloating, mood swings, cramps, weight gain, tender breasts, hot flashes, anxiety and depression, are related to hormonal imbalance, particularly a lack of progesterone. By adding natural progesterone to your system, you achieve the balance that you so desperately need for well-being. I believe that natural progesterone could quite possibly be the antidote for the estrogen overload that we are experiencing.

According to Raymond Peat, M. A., Ph.D., a University of Oregon endocrine physiologist specializing in hormonal changes in stress and aging, progesterone was found to be the basic hormone of adaptation and of resistance to stress. The adrenal glands use it to produce their antistress hormones, and when progesterone is sufficient, they don't have to produce potentially harmful cortisone. In a progesterone deficiency with estrogen dominance, we produce too much cortisone, which causes osteoporosis, aging of the skin, damage to brain cells and accumulation of fat, especially on the back and the abdomen.

Experiments have shown that progesterone relieves anxiety, improves memory and promotes respiration. It reverses many signs of aging and promotes healthy bone growth. It can help to relieve many types of arthritis, and most importantly, it helps a variety of immunological problems. Dr. Peat further recommends that if a woman has ovaries, natural progesterone helps them to produce both progesterone and estrogen as needed and also helps to restore normal functioning of the thyroid and other glands. If a woman's ovaries have been removed, progesterone should be taken consistently to replace the lost supply. A progesterone deficiency has often been associated with an increased susceptibility to cancer.

Progesterone has been used to treat some forms of cancer. When used alone, progesterone often makes it unnecessary to use estrogen for hot flashes, insomnia or other symptoms of menopause. I wholeheartedly agree with Dr. Lee and Dr. Peat. Natural progesterone has been a blessing to the epidemic of hormonal imbalance that women are faced with today. When your body is in balance, your immune system is at its peak. I have developed my own progesterone cream originally out of my own need. Now, many women are enjoying the benefits of natural progesterone across the country. Ordering information can be found at the back of the book.

STRESS AND
YOUR IMMUNE SYSTEM

Peace I leave with you, my peace I give unto you:
not as the world giveth, give I unto you. Let not
your heart be troubled, neither let it be afraid.

—JOHN 14:27

Most of my clients who are chronically ill with lowered immune responses have one thing in common—stress! I have found that in many cases, clients who have been through a stressful period of time in their lives, such as divorce, job loss, sleep deprivation, death in the family, trouble with children and loneliness, have lowered immune responses, which I believe set them up for back-aches, migraines, chronic fatigue syndrome, arthritis, depression, panic disorders, lupus…and the list goes on.

Something else that I have noticed over the past fifteen years is that stress is stress, whether it is good stress or bad stress. Getting married, receiving a job promotion, going on vacation, giving birth, the holidays, moving to a new home or graduating from college or high school are considered happy events in our lives, but there is also a tremendous amount of stress in change—good or bad. I began to notice people with "good" or "bad" stress situations coming down with the same types of chronic illness with lowered immune response. High levels of emotional stress seemed to increase my clients' susceptibility to illness. Also, since stress can lead to suppression of our immune system, it seems that in order to help people overcome their chronic health problems, stress must be dealt with.

God designed our bodies to handle stressful situations.

129

Sometimes we even thrive and are challenged by some of them. Since we can't live in a bubble or run away from all things that upset us, we must maintain a high level of immune health. I believe that illness should not be blamed on stress. I think that we fall victim to stress because of poor health.

The most common causes of stress are emotional and/or physical problems, work addiction, lack of sleep, ingesting too much sugar, caffeine and alcohol, vitamin and mineral depletion from a poor diet, unemployment, marital problems, being a caregiver and hypoglycemia—just to name a few.

In my journey back to health, I was told that the Epstein-Barr virus that I had was usually caused by stress, followed by a lowered immune response. Bingo! They were right. My illness came right after giving birth to my third child, Jillian, who was delivered by cesarean section. Jillian was very sick at birth. In fact, we could have lost her. Then to make matters worse, I hemorrhaged and could not bond with her right away while she was in intensive care. To top this off, this occurred in a hospital six hours away from my home, so I had zero visitors. After returning home, I thought all was well, so I taught aerobics, entertained at retirement homes at night and took care of the house, my husband and children. All of a sudden, wham—illness. I didn't listen to the gentle whispers of the Lord. So He allowed me to go through a wilderness time to de-stress, recover and seek His face.

I had the very same profile that many of my clients have now—a very obvious need for strengthening the immune system. The birth of my child, her illness, my sleep deprivation, demanding workload and poor diet increased my stress levels, which added up to disease. As I tell my clients, "When your body is not at ease mentally, physically or spiritually, then you set yourself up for dis-ease." Try to remember this the next time your stress level is high.

Let me offer some constructive help for handling stress. Believe it or not, some people actually thrive on stress. I have found that these people usually have a few things going for them that chronically stressed, chronically ill people do not. As a rule, they have better coping skills when it comes to stress. This may be due to their prayer life, family support, good friends and the enjoyment of their professions. In addition, they seem to take care of themselves by eating right, getting enough sleep, making time for exercise and having a sense of humor. Where did we hear this before?

> A cheerful heart is good medicine, but a crushed spirit drys up the bones.
>
> —PROVERBS 17:22, NIV

> He leadeth me beside the still waters. He restoreth my soul.
>
> —PSALM 23:2–3

Here is the protocol I used and continue to use to combat stress. I recommend it any time you are dealing with a stressful period. This will keep you strong and well-armed against the many unrelenting problems we face on a daily basis.

HOW TO COMBAT STRESS

Eliminate
- Caffeine
- Sugars
- Colas/soft drinks (these substances will tax the adrenal glands, leaving them weakened and unable to handle stress efficiently)

Diet
- Fresh, whole-food diet moderate in protein, low in fat
- High-complex carbohydrates
- Celery and carrot juice (50/50 mix) as this helps calm nerves, has high mineral and antioxidant content
- Plenty of water

Vitamins and minerals (take daily)
- B-complex vitamin: needed for stress handling; maintains healthy nerves
- Magnesium: relaxes muscles
- Calcium (CalMax formula): helps you sleep; prevents muscle cramps, heart palpitations; helps prevent bone loss
- Pantothenic acid (B_5): rebuilds adrenal glands; antistress vitamin
- ACES: a good antioxidant (Ester C is easier on the digestive system)

Herbs
- Passionflower: for mentally worried and over-tired individuals; helps promote refreshing sleep for emotionally upset; helps relieve irritability with tension
- Reishi mushroom capsules: provides balancing for the entire immune system and has a tonic effect on the whole body system
- Valerian: beneficial for emotional stress and pain. (Do not take if you take antianxiety medication or medicine for depression. If you are pregnant, consult your health care provider on these recommendations.)
- Kava kava (Do not take if you take antianxiety medication or medicine for depression. If you are pregnant, consult your health care provider on these recommendations.)
- Wild American ginseng: adaptogen to help the body deal with stress from physical and emotional imbalance
- Chamomile tea at bed time
- Astragalus: tonic herb for strengthening the immune system.

Body work
- Warm bath before bed with lavender oil
- Consider getting a weekly massage
- Exercise moderately
- Deep breathing—slowly inhale to a count of 4, hold to a count of 4, exhale to a count of 4.

Spirit
- Pray: go deep into the Word of God

Catch stress before it catches you!

Recognizing the early signs of stress and taking action early on to handle it through exercise, relaxation, dietary changes and prayer, rather than letting stress become destructive, will make a difference in your quality of life and well-being. Take this stress-rating quiz.

Stand still, and consider the wondrous works of God.

—Job 37:14

	EVENT VALUE	PT	SCORE
1.	Death of spouse	100	_____
2.	Divorce	78	_____
3.	Marital separation	65	_____
4.	Detention in jail	63	_____
5.	Death of close family member other than spouse	63	_____
6.	Major personal injury or illness	53	_____
7.	Dismissal from job	47	_____
8.	Marriage	50	_____
9.	Marital reconciliation	45	_____
10.	Retirement	45	_____
11.	Major changes in health or behavior in family member	44	_____
12.	Pregnancy	40	_____
13.	Sexual difficulties	39	_____
14.	Major business readjustment	39	_____
15.	Major change in financial status	38	_____
16.	Death of close friend	37	_____
17.	Change in occupation	36	_____
18.	Change in number of arguments with spouse	35	_____
19.	Going into debt for major purchase	31	_____
20.	Foreclosure of mortgage or loan	30	_____
21.	Major change in responsibility at work	29	_____
22.	Son or daughter leaving home for college or marriage	29	_____

	EVENT VALUE	PT	SCORE
23.	Trouble with in-laws	29	_____
24.	Outstanding personal achievement	28	_____
25.	Spouse begins or ceases work outside the home	26	_____
26.	Beginning or ceasing formal schooling	26	_____
27.	Major change in living conditions, for example, new home, remodeling	25	_____
28.	Revision of personal habits	24	_____
29.	Trouble with your boss	23	_____
30.	Major change in working hours or conditions	20	_____
31.	Change in residence	20	_____
32.	Change in schools	20	_____
33.	Major change in usual type or amount of recreation	19	_____
34.	Major change in church activities	18	_____
35.	Taking a loan out for smaller purchases	17	_____
36.	Major change in social activities	18	_____
37.	Major change in sleeping habits	16	_____
38.	Major change in family get-togethers	15	_____
39.	Major change in eating habits	15	_____
40.	Vacation	13	_____
41.	Christmas/holiday season	12	_____
42.	Minor legal violations	11	_____

TOTAL

STRESS RATING SCALE

A score below 150 points means statistically that you have a 30 percent chance of developing a significant health problem in the near future. A score between 150 and 300 points gives you a 50 percent chance of developing a significant health problem. A score of more than 300 points raises the possibility of a significant health problem to a whopping 80 percent.

The stress scale quiz shows you that stress is indeed cumulative. The good news is that by implementing methods for coping with stress, you do not have to become a statistic but an overcomer. The key is to recognize and diffuse your stress before this ticking time bomb explodes and you are faced with a serious health problem. In the 90-Day Immune System Makeover, I have given you most of the earthly tools known for stress management. Of course, you know that your best stress weapon is to cast all your cares upon the Lord. Do it daily. Do it minute by minute if you have to. But do it. He will see you through. He will not fail you, because He cannot.

Four indicators of stress

> I will give peace...and none shall make you afraid.
>
> —LEVITICUS 26:6

1. Sagging of the corners of the eyes, having a short temper, nervousness, creases in the forehead, irritability
2. Fatigue, anger, insomnia, impatience, sadness, crying, overreacting
3. Chronic neck or back pain, headaches, high blood pressure, stomach problems, accelerated aging
4. Frequent infections, asthma, heart disease, mental or emotional breakdown, kidney malfunction

If you can relate to any of the four indicators above, you must take steps to de-stress. A constant state of distress can wreak havoc on your immune system. Because stress can alter the body's chemical balance, it has a direct influence on the development of many diseases.

For as [a man] thinks in his heart, so is he.

—Proverbs 23:7, NKJV

When it comes to the dynamics of stress, your thoughts are the key. What you think can literally make you sick or healthy. If you continually dwell on the past and what could have been or should have been, or if you hold on to anger or unforgiveness, the result will be the production of large amounts of adrenaline and other powerful chemicals from your internal pharmacy. Long-term manufacture and release of these strong substances can eventually lead to heart disease, ulcer, high blood pressure and cancer.

You must flood your body with good memories of happy times. Forgive others who have hurt you, and let go of anger as if it were a helium-filled balloon that you release into a bright blue sky. This will encourage your internal pharmacy to release pain-relieving, mood-lifting, immune-strengthening endorphins. Proper endorphin levels can make the immune system run like a high-performance engine. They even chase after harmful substances in your body.

It seems logical now that higher endorphin levels are what you should aim for...but how? It is said that one of the best ways to raise endorphin levels is to be in love with someone, something, an idea or a cause. The happy, positive feeling of being in love increases your level of endorphins and makes you feel wonderful while strengthening your immune system.

In his book *Health in the 21st Century: Will Doctors Survive?*, Dr. Francisco Contreras wrote about The Menninger Clinic of Topeka, Kansas, and its studies on love. It was found that people in love have lower levels of lactic acid in the bloodstream, which causes them to feel less tired and have higher levels of endorphins. In turn, they feel euphoric and less sensitive to pain. In addition, their white corpuscles respond better to infection and they catch fewer colds.

Exercise is also an effective way to raise endorphin levels. A good workout can have beneficial effects. One word of caution: In many stressed people, I have found that A-type personalities, that is, go all out or not at all, seem to overexercise, further stressing their systems. There must be a total shift in your thinking. Moderation is key. According to John Hibbs, N.D., of Bastyr College in Seattle, Washington, "I don't think there's a single thing in life as therapeutic as the right kind of exercise program applied over a period of time. But misapplied it can be just another stressor." I couldn't agree more.

Stress: The natural approach

Daniel O. Gagnon, a medical herbalist, recommends chamomile to promote relaxation. I agree. Chamomile has been used by millions of people for generations to promote relaxation. Another benefit is that it soothes gastritis, which often goes hand in hand with stress. Gagnon also recommends American ginseng, which "helps the body be more prepared and more resistant to everyday stresses."

Of course, proper nutrition is crucial in keeping your body armed against the effects of stress. As your stress level increases, protein needs go up. I remember hearing years ago that when you are under extreme stress, the amount of protein used in one day is equal to the protein in one gallon of milk! Try adding these protein foods when under stress: whole grains, fresh seafood (white fish, no scavengers), soy foods, eggs, carrot juice and green vegetables. In the following pages, I'll have a more complete protocol.

Pause here for a stressbuster

Take a rest and relaxation period every day. Listen to soft, beautiful music. Afterward, take three minutes to systematically tense and relax every muscle from the top of your head to the soles of your feet. Meditate on the scriptures throughout this book.

> God is not the author of confusion but of peace.
> —1 Corinthians 14:33, NKJV

Your "MANTLE" for stress relief

I have found in my own life that when I am faced with stress and tension, my muscles tighten all over my body, and I generally feel miserable. I began research into muscle tension and found that physical and emotional stress gets stored in your muscles, making you even more tense. Fortunately, there are solutions when you feel yourself tightening up. Massage therapy has a long history of therapeutic benefits. A stressed body responds beautifully to regular massage therapy sessions. If this sounds a bit unpractical for you, do not worry; there is always exercise, like walking, stretching and light weightlifting. But I want to share with you a wonderful technique that will work for you time and time again when you are faced with a body that is tight with stressed muscles. I call it the "MANTLE technique." I continue to use it even as I am writing this book to relieve the tightness in my neck and shoulders. It is very simple. My MANTLE technique is simply tensing and holding for the count of ten each part of your body, one section at a time. To remind myself that I need attention daily, I thought of the word mantle.

M—Muscles
A—always
N—need
T—tension
L—loosening
E—every day.

That's right; muscles always need tension loosening every day. Begin with your eyes: Tense and hold for ten seconds, then release. Take a deep, cleansing breath. Try to belly breathe. (Fill your diaphragm with air and exhale slowly through your mouth.) Next, tighten all of the muscles of your face and mouth; make a face and hold it for ten seconds. Take another deep, cleansing breath. Continue this tensing and releasing exercise on down to the other parts of your body. This would include your neck, shoulders, arms, hands, fingers, stomach, lower abdomen, upper thighs, calves, feet and toes. After each area has been relaxed, give thanks to God for all of His wonderful blessings He has bestowed upon you, and give Him praise for them all.

Great is the LORD and greatly to be praised.
—1 CHRONICLES 16:25

Quick relaxer
To ease your neck muscles, place your thumbs at the

base of your skull, just below your ears. Press inward and upward for six seconds, then release. Repeat, moving your thumbs a quarter-inch inward along the base of your skull each time.

To relax your lower back, put four tennis balls in a sock. Place the sock at the base of your back, lie down on them, and roll gently for a few minutes. Your body weight applies the pressure.

To relax your shoulders, place your fingertips on your shoulders at the base of your neck. Press down, holding the pressure for six seconds. Release, then repeat, gradually working your fingers down your shoulder line.

The fight-or-flight response

Here is a summary of what happens when you experience stress. The rate of your breathing increases to supply necessary oxygen to the heart. The heart rate and the force of contraction of the heart increase to provide more blood to the muscles and brain. The liver dumps more stored glucose into the bloodstream to energize the body to begin physical activity. Sweat production increases to eliminate toxic compounds produced by the body and to lower body temperature.

Here is the relaxation response in summary. The heart rate and blood pressure are reduced. The rate of breathing decreases because oxygen demand is reduced when a person is relaxed. The stomach produces more hydrochloric acid, which in turn aids in digestion. The liver secretes less glucose, and blood sugar levels are reduced. You can see it is desirable to live in a relaxed state where your body is not working overtime. In order to achieve this, you must exercise and use nutrition and nutritional therapies as outlined in the makeover program. Practice the MANTLE technique, commonly called progressive relaxation, and finally, focus on God, not on your problems.

The new frontier of medicine: The mind

Between 60 and 90 percent of all medical office visits in the United States are for stress-related disorders, according to The Mind/Body Medical Institute at Harvard Medical School.

Mind/body medicine is based on thousands of studies over the past twenty-five years and is now considered mainstream. The use of relaxation techniques to fight stress-related illnesses could be one of the most important medical treatments of the twenty-first century. Dr. Gregg D. Jacobs, an assistant professor of psychiatry at Harvard Medical School and a senior scientist with the Mind/Body Institute, discussed at the Medicine in the Millennium Conference that there is a proven link between thoughts and emotions and the health of the body. In addition to good nutrition and exercise, practicing the relaxation response makes your cells that fight disease more effective. The relaxation response involves changing one's thoughts, which in turn lowers the body's metabolism, heart rate, breathing rate and blood pressure. It has also been shown to improve a person's sense of well-being. The relaxation response can be achieved through progressive muscle relaxation, focused breathing, music or prayer. It is cost effective with little or no side effects, and the techniques can be taught through books or tapes.

While I am on the subject of stress, I would be remiss if I did not discuss at length the importance of the B vitamins. Proper functioning of the nervous system is affected by the B vitamins. I believe that B vitamins are the most influential factor in maintaining a healthy nervous system. When my clients are under stress of any kind, whether it be physical, emotional or mental, I recommend a good total B-complex post haste. As you read on, you will see why the B vitamins are my favorite in times of stress.

Thiamine, or B_1, is known as the "morale vitamin" because of its beneficial effect on mental attitude. It is also crucial to the health of the nervous system. If your diet is high in carbohydrates, then B_1 is absolutely essential. B_1 also improves food assimilation, thereby stabilizing your appetite. Here are the symptoms of B_1 deficiency: fatigue, loss of ankle and knee reflexes, mental instability, forgetfulness, fears, inflammation of the optic nerve and cardiac malfunctions such as rapid rhythm and palpitations.

Riboflavin, or Vitamin B_2, is also a water-soluble vitamin that is easily absorbed through the small intestine. It plays an important part in any chemical reactions in the body. B_2 deficiency symptoms are as follows: shiny tongue, burning and itching eyes, feeling of sand or grit in eyes, oily skin, difficulty in urination and scaling around mouth, nose and ears. B_2 has aso been shown to be an inhibitor of tumor growth.

B_6 seems to have the greatest effect on the immune system of all the B vitamins because a deficiency can result in a vast array of problems in the immune response. A lack of B_6 will decrease the size of the thymus gland, which produces T cells. A deficiency of B_6 also relates to tumor growth.

B_{12} is a B vitamin that neither man nor animal can manufacture in their bodies. Also known as cobalamin, it is the most complex molecularly of all the B vitamins. The largest amounts of B_{12} are found in brewer's yeast, eggs, clams, herring, kidney, liver and milk and dairy products. Vegetarians need to make sure their intake of B_{12} is sufficient by eating soy, kelp and soybeans because animal sources supply most of the B_{12} our body needs. A B-complex vitamin will ensure that you are covering all the B-vitamin bases.

B_{12} is needed in the body for the formation of red blood cells. B_{12} must be combined with calcium for proper absorption. B_{12} has a stimulating effect on the immune system. When deficient T and B cell responses diminish, pernicious anemia may occur, along with sore tongue, weight loss, mental deterioration, menstrual disturbances and "needles and pins" sensation.

Pantothenic acid, or B_5, is a blessing when a person is under stress. It remains my favorite even now. It has an enhancing and beneficial effect upon the adrenal glands where proper functioning is crucial during times of stressful conditions.

With this information in mind, be sure to take your B vitamins.

PRAYER AND IMMUNITY

Is prayer good for your body as well as your soul? Many studies are now showing that people who regularly attend prayer services tend to be in better health and live longer than people who rarely set foot in a house of prayer. Some skeptics believe that this is because churchgoers generally have fewer vices, which makes them fitter. To see if this theory held any water, epidemiologist William Strawbridge from the Public Health Institute did a study over three decades of five thousand Christians from California, some practicing, some not. His study showed that church devotees who attended church once a week or more had lower death rates than those who attended occasionally if at all. He also noted that church members who started off with bad health habits such as smoking and alcohol tended to give up these vices, whether from peer pressure or simply being observant of their faith. In conclusion, Strawbridge believes that there is no denying that faithful church attendance enhances a person's sense of belonging and well-being. This in turn boosts immunity. Those of us who are believers agree 100 percent.

WHAT DOES THE BIBLE SAY ABOUT STRESS, FEAR AND ANXIETY?

Therefore I tell you, do not be anxious about your life, what you shall eat or what you shall drink, nor about your body, what you shall put on. Is not life more than food, and the body more than clothing? Look at the birds of the air; they neither sow nor reap nor gather into barns, and yet your heavenly Father feeds them. Are you not of more value than they? And which of you by being anxious can add one cubit to his life span? . . . Therefore do not be anxious, saying, "What shall we eat?" or "What shall we drink?" or "What shall we wear?" For the Gentiles seek all these things; and your heavenly

Father knows that you need them all. But seek first his kingdom and his righteousness, and all these things shall be yours as well. Therefore do not be anxious about tomorrow, for tomorrow will be anxious for itself. Let the days own trouble be sufficient for the day.

—MATTHEW 6:25–27, 31–34, RSV

The Bible teaches us that we should not be anxious, fearful or stressed if we put our faith and trust in Christ. If you are dealing with stress and anxiety in your life, read this scripture daily. Jesus lived in stressful times that were filled with fear and anxiety. How did Jesus deal with His anxious moments? He knew how to carry everything to His Father and leave it there. God is your Father also. Every day, immediately go to the Father in confidence and prayer when you are anxious, fearful or stressed. The Word of God sustains us more than any health food, vitamin or herbal program. God will keep your mind from anxiety, fear and stress if you commune with Him daily. God is in charge; He is on the throne. Carry your troubles to Him. He will demonstrate His love for you. People who suffer from anxiety seem to feel all alone and hopeless. He will be there to protect you, guide you and give you His peace. He is right beside you always, having your best interest at heart.

For a more in-depth study concerning God's provision for healing from stress and all of its resultant afflictions, read this following section by Pastor John Jeyaseelan. You will find that he truly knows the power of God's promise of healing and restoration through prayer. I am blessed to have found such a wonderful ministry with which to partner. During some of my most stressful times, John and his wife, Hema, have kept me in prayer. They continue to support prayerfully every area of my life. I am sure you will be blessed and your immune makeover enhanced by the following words from John:

PRAYER SUPPORT FROM JOHN JEYASEELAN

Scripture teaches us that healing will often follow God's forgiveness in our lives. King David enjoyed the fruits of prayer and praise to his God, and he commanded his soul to remember what the Lord had done:

> Bless the LORD, O my soul: and all that is within me, bless his holy name. Bless the LORD, O my soul, and forget not all his benefits: who forgiveth all thine iniquities; who healeth all thy diseases; who redeemeth thy life from destruction; who crowneth thee with lovingkindness and tender mercies; who satisfieth thy mouth with good things, so that thy youth is renewed like the eagle's.
> —PSALM 103:1–5

At another time, King David cried out to God to restore the joy of his salvation after repenting for his sin with Bathsheba:

> Have mercy upon me, O God, according to thy lovingkindness; according unto the multitude of thy tender mercies blot out my transgressions. Wash me throughly from mine iniquity, and cleanse me from my sin. For I acknowledge my transgressions: and my sin is ever before me...Restore unto me the

joy of thy salvation; and uphold me with thy free
spirit.

—Psalm 51:1–3,12

The stress related to David's sin and guilt was dealt
with after an honest prayer of confession and repentance
to God. Only then could God restore the joy in David's
life.

Like David, my healing came as a result of my direct
experience with God after confessing my sins and
vowing to change my life.

This section focuses on healing and health as a result
of our walk and prayerful communication with God.
God made you a whole person!

God created man in His own image and gave him a
spirit, soul and body. In His Word, He has also given us
clear instructions for the maintenance of our spirits,
our souls and our bodies.

> And God said, Let us make man in our image,
> after our likeness: and let them have dominion
> over the fish of the sea, and over the fowl of the
> air, and over the cattle, and over all the earth. . . .
> So God created man in his own image, in the
> image of God created he him; male and female
> created he them.
>
> —GENESIS 1:26–27

> And the LORD God formed man of the dust of the
> ground, and breathed into his nostrils the breath
> of life; and man became a living soul.
>
> —GENESIS 2:7

The above passages tell how God created man as a
whole being. Any instruction to improving the body's

147

immune system cannot be complete if it is limited to only medicine and nutrition for the physical body. This approach ignores one-third of our being. Man's spiritual condition must also be addressed.

God's instruction to Adam and Eve concerning the forbidden fruit was clear:

> In the day that thou eatest thereof thou shalt die.
> —GENESIS 2:17

When man sinned, death came as a curse. Just as death came as a curse resulting from man breaking the law, the word of God, life and health are man's reward when we obey the Living Word of God, Jesus Christ.

Christ came in obedience to the mission of God, to seek and save the lost. Jesus committed Himself to fulfill all righteousness at the Jordan and yielded His body and will to the mission of the cross. Christ is the Savior of the whole man: the spirit, the soul and the body. When we come to Christ, we receive eternal life. Eternal life, contrary to popular belief, does not start at the moment of death but at the moment of our rebirth in Christ.

Death is merely the removal of the limitations of our physical body, which allows us to move to a higher level of eternal life. However, our quality of overall life and our health rise to new dimensions with our dependence on God's Word to daily guide us through every aspect of life. Like Jesus, we must also give the whole man to the obedience of God's work.

It was through Christ and His obedience that the curse of the law (poverty, sickness and death) was broken: "Christ hath redeemed us from the curse of the law, being made a curse for us: for it is written, Cursed is everyone that hangeth on a tree" (Gal. 3:13).

Some of the sicknesses that resulted from breaking God's law are listed in Deuteronomy 12: boils, pestilence, tumors, scab, itch, madness, blindness, heart problems, arthritis, cancer and continuously clinging sicknesses. When we walk daily in Christ and in obedience to the Word of God, we share in the fruits of the broken curse: health and wellness. God promises healing in His Word!

God said to Israel:

> If thou wilt diligently hearken to the voice of the LORD thy God, and wilt do that which is right in his sight, and wilt give ear to his commandments, and keep all his statutes, I will put none of the diseases upon thee, which I have brought upon the Egyptians: for I am the LORD that healeth thee.
>
> —EXODUS 15:26

Healing and deliverance are promised to the believer through the redeeming and atoning blood shed by Jesus on the cross. Healing and health are promised to those who pray to the Lord:

> Is any sick among you? Let him call for the elders of the church; and let them pray over him, anointing him with oil in the name of the Lord: and the prayer of faith shall save the sick, and the Lord shall raise him up.
>
> —JAMES 5:14–15

Jesus carried our sicknesses and pain upon His body.

> Surely he hath borne our griefs [sicknesses], and carried our sorrows [pains]: yet we did esteem him stricken, smitten of God, and afflicted. But he was wounded for our transgressions, he was bruised

for our iniquities: the chastisement of our peace
was upon him; and with his stripes we are healed.

—ISAIAH 53:4–5

When Israel prayed to God, the Bible tells us that
"[God] sent his word, and healed them, and delivered
them from their destructions"(Ps. 107:20).

There is divine healing when a believer prays! Healing
is part of the atonement in God's Word. God is not only
able but also willing to heal the one who calls upon His
name. Remember the blind beggar Bartimaeus who
called upon the name of Jesus repeatedly to get His
attention. When he did, Jesus healed him. Jesus respects
faith, and when we call on Him with the faith of
Bartimaeus, He will listen to our cry and bring healing to
our lives.

My first major healing came as a result of my grandmother's prayers two years before my bout with peptic
ulcers. (Unfortunately, I did not learn from it). I was
seventeen years old and suffering from tuberculosis.
After three months with the disease and losing much
weight, I was admitted to the hospital. The doctors who
examined me found that more than half of my lungs
were infected with TB, and I was immediately quaran-
tined. None of family were allowed to see me. Those
were horrible days for me. I was very frightened!

However, unknown to me, my godly grandmother
was in constant prayer for me. As I found out later, her
prayer was simple and straightforward: "Lord Jesus, I
am sixty-five years old, and there is not much I can do
for You. Plant my life into my grandson; heal him of this
deadly disease so that he can live to tell the world that
You are true to Your Word and that You answer
prayers."

She kept repeating this prayer over and over again from my home, which was fifty miles away from the hospital. God heard her cry and answered her prayers. There was a miraculous recovery in my body, and on the tenth day of my quarantine, x-rays showed me free of any tuberculosis. The doctors were shocked and amazed!

On my return home my grandmother hugged me and related to me how Jesus had answered her prayers. He also told her she would be home with Him in heaven the following year. Indeed, my grandmother died the following year with great anticipation and excitement in her heart. It was much later in life that I learned that God's Word tells us that He answers the prayers of His loved ones: "Is any sick among you? Let him call for the elders of the church; and let them pray over him, anointing him with oil in the name of the Lord; and the prayer of faith shall save the sick, and the Lord shall raise him up; and if he have committed sins, they shall be forgiven him. Confess your faults one to another, and pray one for another, that ye may be healed. The effectual fervent prayer of a righteous man availeth much" (James 5:14–16).

Imagine a healthy life through prayer and walking with God! God promised us a healthy life if we follow Him. God's promise to His people is made abundantly clear in His Word: "Ye shall observe to do therefore as the LORD your God hath commanded you: ye shall not turn aside to the right hand or to the left. Ye shall walk in all the ways which the LORD your God hath commanded you, that ye may live, and that it may be well with you, and that ye may prolong your days in the land which ye shall possess" (Deut. 5:32–33).

Many believers pay little attention to God's promises

according to His covenant in the Old Testament, giving credence only to His promises in the New Testament. This attitude is in direct opposition to Hebrews 13:8:

> Jesus Christ the same yesterday, and to day, and for ever.

Jesus Christ was the Living Word of God long before the New Testament was written. Whether in the Old or the New Testament, by faith you can stand on God's promises.

Start a consistent daily prayer life! The Bible tells us to "pray without ceasing" (1 Thess. 5:17). An ounce of prevention is worth a pound of cure. The following are examples found in God's Word urging the preparation of our spirit with a consistent prayer life and its corresponding benefits:

Jesus encouraged His disciples to enter into an hour of prayer with Him so that they "enter not into temptation" (Matt. 26:40–41). An hour of prayer every day in the presence of God will keep you from the temptations of the world.

The apostle James writes that "every man is tempted, when he is drawn away of his own lust, and enticed" (James 1:14). Daily prayer keeps you away from temptations, lusts, sin and their consequences, which include stress and sickness.

Before entering into the Promised Land, God admonished the people of Israel to set aside a day to sanctify themselves, for the Lord would do wonders among them the following day (Josh. 3:1–5). A day of fasting and prayer from time to time cleanses our system and prepares us to retain the blessings of God in our lives, which include our health.

Three days of entering into God's presence changes your destiny.

Abraham's three-day walk in obedience to God's command to sacrifice his son, Isaac, brought him into his destiny as "father of many nations."

Jonah was in the belly of the fish three days, crying out to God, to complete his destiny of turning Nineveh to revival.

The apostle Paul was struck with blindness for three days before yielding to the call of God in his life (Acts 9:9–16). When a life-threatening situation confronts us, it is good to withdraw from all negative inputs and concentrate on God's Word in prayer to boost our hope and see reversal in most situations.

Seven days of staying in the presence of God in prayer completes that which God begins in you.

David sought the Lord for forgiveness of the sin with Bathsheba and the child born in sin. While the child died, God forgave David and brought Solomon ("Jedidiah," "beloved of Jehovah") into his life and restored the joy of David's salvation (2 Sam. 12:16–18, 24–25). David was free from the guilt and stress caused by his violation of God's law. According to The Mind/Body Medical Institute at Harvard Medical School, between 60 and 90 percent of all medical office visits in the United States are for stress-related disorders.

Ten days of prayer while waiting on God's promises will bring fulfillment of that same promise.

The disciples waited in the upper room in the presence of God for ten days to receive the promised Holy Spirit (Acts 2:1–4). When the Spirit of God nudges us to wait on Him for a few days or for a few weeks for an answer, we must obey and never lose faith. We must never give up! The Amplified Bible translates Matthew 7:7 as follows: "Keep on asking and it will be given you; keep on seeking and you will find; keep on knocking [reverently] and [the door] will be opened to you." We must keep on asking and seeking until the Spirit of God releases us from doing so.

Twenty-one days of fasting and prayer by Daniel brought him the latter-day revelations from God (Dan. 10:2–21). As a result of my recent fasting and prayer of twenty-one days, not only did I lose a few pounds but I emerged from it full of both physical and spiritual energy. (Warning: If you have never fasted before, do not attempt more than one or two days of fasting without consulting your physician. Certainly, do not attempt twenty-one days of fasting.)

Forty days of walking with God in His presence alters history. Moses was in the presence of God's glory for forty days and received the Law, which altered the Jewish way of life and paved the way for Christian living (Exod. 24:15–18). Jonah cried out against Nineveh for forty days before the revival came upon that nation. After forty days, Elijah received directions concerning the leadership of Syria, Israel and his own successor, Elisha. Forty days of fasting and prayer empowered Jesus with the power and the anointing of the Holy Spirit to enable Him to do what He was sent to do, to bring salvation to the world.

God will most assuredly change the direction of your life as a result of your constant prayer, thus avoiding the pitfalls of wrong and erroneous decisions and their consequences.

Three months of prayer and abiding in God's glorious presence changes your life forever. Obededom is the prime example of this. (See 2 Samuel 6:11.) You will most certainly see such a difference God has made in your life in ninety days as a result of prayer and walking with God that you will keep it the most important priority every day of your life.

In the above passages, we have seen how a consistent prayer life, starting with an hour every day for up to ninety days, cleanses you from guilt, anxiety, stress and gives you clear direction through the counsel and guidance of God in your life. You will enjoy a life of freedom and liberty in Christ. It is amazing that in ninety days, a godly habit of praying and yielding to God's will in your life begins to take effect. As God ordained seasons in nature such as springtime and harvest, you too will come into a season of prayer and harvesting the principles and benefits of godly living. Your daily prayer should include the following:

1. Adoring God and His attributes
2. Confessing of His lordship over you
3. Thanking Him for all answers to prayers in the past
4. Reminding Him of His promises and provisions in your life
5. Confessing your sin to God and receiving forgiveness from Him
6. Seeking counsel concerning every situation or matter in your life
7. Being honest to reveal your hurts and pains and believing in faith for answers
8. Forgiving those who wronged you—prayer without forgiveness will not bless you
9. Praying with humbleness of heart—without humility there will be no healing

10. Listening to God's direction through the unction of His Spirit—God does speak to all His children
11. If you are certain that God has commanded you to take certain steps or actions, then do so in full obedience. Remember, God will never ask you or direct you to do or say anything that is contrary to His Word
12. Fulfilling all vows you make to God. It is better not to vow than to vow and then renege.

Do this consistently for ninety days. In addition to praying alone, join with your family and other support groups from your church, and pray corporately on a regular basis. You will then come into a comfortable rhythm of praying and walking with God. By the end of this period, you will have experienced heavenly provisions for your health and joy. The atmosphere at home will change so rapidly that you will enjoy God's presence for the rest of your life just as Obededom did! Then of course, continue to pray and walk with Christ all of your life.

Dearly beloved, as you purpose to seek the Lord with all your heart and mind daily and follow a healthy regimen concerning nutrition and physical well-being, God will keep sickness and disease out of your life with an added spiritual immune system that protects the whole person...body, soul and spirit. May the Lord bless you with His health today and always.

STRESSED OUT?
GRAB SOME GABA

You are now going to learn about an amino acid that

has shown excellent results in treating anxiety, depression, brain and nerve dysfunctions, extreme nervous tension, insomnia, high blood pressure, schizophrenia, Parkinson's disease and Alzheimer's disease. This marvelous amino acid is known as gamma-aminobutyric acid, or GABA. GABA acts as one of the nervous system's neurotransmitters. It helps to inhibit nerve cells from overfiring, thereby preventing anxiety and stress from wreaking havoc on the brain. It does this by filling brain receptors that become depleted during long or intense periods of stress. The exciting news is that GABA has been shown to be as effective as pharmaceutical anxiety medications such as Valium, Xanax and Ativan. More importantly, the risk of addiction does not exist with GABA as with current anxiety medications.

You may have noticed that in many health food stores, whole sections are dedicated to stress, sleep and relaxation formulas. Pick up one of those formulas, and you will notice that almost every one of them contains GABA. Supplement companies always stay current and on the cutting edge with their formulations. It is their business to do so. It is common knowledge to them that GABA has shown very promising results in returning anxiety-ridden individuals to their former selves. Best of all, GABA may prevent individuals from living their lives in the "chemical straight jacket" provided by anxiety medications. Other uses for GABA include treatment for attention deficit hyperactivity disorder, or ADHD, and hypertension, primarily because of its relaxant properties. Billie Jay Sahley, Ph.D., has authored several books on anxiety and emotional healing and the use of amino acid therapy as an alternative to prescription anxiety medication. Her work is birthed out of her own struggle with panic and anxiety disorder.

The goal of this makeover program is to give you as much information as I possibly can to help you live a higher quality of life. Like Billie Jay Sahley, I too suffered with panic attacks that were so frightening and disabling that sometimes it was hard to go on with my life. It was a lonely walk, but out of it came the knowledge of what to do and how to regain a sense of normalcy once again. Prayers are answered and sent perhaps through a person, book, magazine or documentary. God will send you an answer to whatever you are facing. In the case of panic attacks, Dr. Sahley's wonderful books started my journey back from the abyss of anxiety. If you scored high on the stress scale, consider taking GABA before you get as depleted as I was. Experts recommend that you find a formula with GABA, inositol and niacinamide for a synergistic, more effective formula. For a more in-depth study into GABA and other amino acids for the relief of anxiety, I highly recommend that you read *The Anxiety Epidemic* by Billie Jay Sahley, Ph.D. It is available from Pain and Stress Publications, San Antonio, Texas. You call 1-800-669-CALM.

EIGHT STRESSBUSTERS TO BOOST IMMUNITY

A certain level of stress is not only normal, but it is an expected part of life. Only when stress is severe, long lasting or happens frequently will our health be jeopardized.

1. *Eat well.* Eating right will keep you well enough to face distressing challenges.
2. *Sleep deep.* Sleeping soundly is essential for a continually healthy immune system.
3. *Confide in a friend.* In times of great stress, you need to be able to talk about your problem and discuss its details with a person you trust and who has concern for you.
4. *Express yourself.* Verbalization of your problem has long been recognized by the psychological sciences as an effective tool for releasing the tensions of those problems that result in stress.
5. *Get physical.* The movement of blood increases general immune protection and at the same time helps buffer the immunosuppression of distress. Regular exercise is a natural release for the body's response to stress.
6. *Time to unwind.* Have a relaxation period set aside each day to listen to music, take a warm bath, take up a hobby, take a private walk or practice deep breathing. Pick the activity that leaves you feeling refreshed, renewed and rejuvenated.
7. *Remain clear-headed.* Alcohol or drugs will not cure distress. Your immune system is already suppressed by stress and becomes more so by alcohol or drug use.
8. *Pray.* Give your cares and worries to the Lord.

60-DAY RECOMMENDED SUPPLEMENTS

- CalMax powder

Natural antibiotics (if needed, choose one at a time):
- Biotic silver
- Olive leaf extract
- Grapefruit seed extract
- Oil of oregano
- Goldenseal
- Garlic

Essential fatty acids (choose one):
- Nature's Secret Ultimate Oil
- Carlson's Salmon Oil
- Kyolic-EPA
- Flaxseed oil

Probiotics:
- Kyo-Dophilus by Wakunaga
- Acidophilus bifidus formula

Plant enzymes: (choose the formula that fits your profile)
- Enzymedica Plant Enzyme Formulas (Lipo, Gastro, Digest or Purify)

Fiber supplement (if needed):
- Nature's Secret Ultimate Fiber

Candida control product:
- Candistroy by Nature's Secret

Adrenal gland health:
- Astragalus
- Pantothenic acid, 500 mg.
- Royal jelly
- Adrenal gland supplement

Hormonal balance
- Progesterone cream
- Dr. Janet's Balanced by Nature Progesterone Cream

Stress (if not on medication, try these one at a time):
- Kava kava
- Chamomile tea
- Reishi mushroom
- Valerian
- Passionflower
- GABA

PART THREE:

90 Days

---■---

90 Days

You did it! You have completed the 90-Day Immune System Makeover. You have boosted your immune health by eliminating from your diet and lifestyle all of the major causes of disease and sub-health in our time. By doing this, you have increased your chances of a longer, more vital life. By now you should be feeling better and healthier than you have in many years. You should be calmer, feel stronger, have more energy and be filled with optimism about the future. As I promised, it really has not been that hard to accomplish. God made our bodies wonderfully forgiving, just as He is. You now understand how your body responds to correct dietary, mental and spiritual principals. Most of all, you have learned that good health should not be a struggle.

We are supposed to be healthy. It is our natural state of being. Man has once again gotten in the way of what God has originally planned for us by perverting the

165

food supply, twisting the Word of God and making mankind feel like a failure if certain material things are not obtained or impossible goals accomplished. You now know the truth, and the truth has made you free.

You are probably wondering if the way that you feel right now will last. The answer is yes—if you continue to follow the basic guidelines that I have taught you throughout the makeover process. Most of my clients never want to go back to the way they were before the program. They do not want to revisit all of the troubling symptoms that once interfered with the quality of their lives and affected their relationships with those whom they love.

It is true that there will be times you will revert back to your old ways; after all, you are human. I am way ahead of you here. I have factored this into the 90-Day Immune System Makeover program. I'll tell you now that if you continue on this program only 80 percent, you will still maintain the benefits. Most clients notice an almost immediate return of complaints if they drop under 80 percent compliance. See for yourself. Your body will let you know when you are falling away from the correct path.

I am not saying that you need to be fanatical. What I am saying is that it is perfectly all right to allow yourself to indulge. Just be careful and recognize that oftentimes one indulgence leads to overindulgence, and before you know it, you're back into your old disease-promoting habits that prompted you to begin this program in the first place.

Here are some tips that I give my clients after their makeover: Caffeine, sugar, alcohol, exercise and stress control and smoking must continually be addressed.

Caffeine. Now that you have eliminated caffeine from your life, I am sure that you are doing just fine without it. You may have experienced the headache that often accompanies caffeine withdrawal during elimination. You now know that a substance that causes withdrawal symptoms once you discontinue it is nothing more than a drug. If you do find yourself at a social gathering and feel that you must have a cup of coffee to be "social," then the after effects—feeling anxious and edgy—will be proof enough that you need never to do it again.

In addition, you may feel an energy slump a few hours after that cup of coffee and also have trouble sleeping that night. Most of my clients agree that one caffeine experience after having completed the makeover convinces them to stay away from it for good. They simply want to keep their higher level of health and the pure, clean, natural energy that comes from a balanced system.

Sugar. Sugar is also gladly avoided by clients after the makeover program because they simply do not crave it anymore. In addition, sweet things taste too sweet and have no appeal. Blood sugar levels have become stable, and doughnut, cakes and pastries have lost their appeal. This has strengthened your will power. I recommend that you try to stay away from sugar indefinitely. It is all right, however, to enjoy a piece of birthday cake or wedding cake to celebrate life's special moments. You will be amazed that your desire and taste for that cake will not be as strong as it once was. After one or two bites, the sugary taste will be too much for your tastebuds. You have developed a new taste for whole, health-building foods. Sugar only takes away from your vitality.

Alcohol. Alcohol avoidance is also recommended from now on. One or two glasses of wine or liquor will produce ramifications the next morning. Usually the fatigue, sluggishness and headache simply are not worth it to my clients who have rebuilt their bodies. In essence, they do not want to risk doing anything to jeopardize their state of optimal health. I am not saying a glass of wine once in a while has negative consequences. However, some people simply do not know when to stop. So why take the risk? While one or two glasses of wine a week may not be harmful, more than that can be. Remember, you do not want to reverse your results. You want to move forward to a higher level mentally, physically and spiritually daily. "Always forward, never back, and in your health you'll never lack." This is a little phrase I thought of while I was on my journey to wellness. It kept me on the right path in difficult times. Remember it when you are tempted to tear down your system with dead foods, alcohol, caffeine and sugar.

Exercise and stress control. Exercise should be a permanent part of your life now. You probably have discovered that the more you exercise, the better you feel. The better you feel, the stronger and leaner you become. As an added benefit and a double bonus, you are relieving stress at the same time. You may find after incorporating some form of daily exercise into your life that you no longer have a problem sleeping, focusing or concentrating. Your mind is clearer and your stress levels are lower.

While we are on the subject of stress, keep my MANTLE technique in mind when you do have occasional tension. I practice every day just to give my system a check. It will immediately notify you as to where you are storing stress. I use the technique to relax the entire body, one muscle group at a time, from top to bottom. And of course, practice your deep breathing daily.

Smoking. If you have stopped smoking, congratulations! Did you know that your body has already begun to recover from the negative effects of smoking on your health? At this 90-day mark, you have greatly reduced your risk for tobacco-related disease with your new lifestyle in place. Health was never improved by smoking. If you have not stopped smoking completely, stay in prayer and continue to cut back, and you will overcome and be free of the nicotine habit. Some people lose the desire for a cigarette quickly while others take a few months. Do not compare yourself to others. This is your own walk into vibrant health. Enjoy the process that will continue after these 90-days if you do not look back. Ask your physician for help if you are really struggling. The key is do not give up. You will have the victory.

What I especially find rewarding is the newfound confidence that my clients have when they complete the 90-day makeover. They have a greater appreciation for their health. They know how it feels to feel healthy, and they know what to do to stay that way. They feel empowered with the knowledge they have acquired to overcome the attack upon their physical bodies. They now feel that they can fulfill the divine purpose God has given them. They have a renewed zest for life and a spirit of sharing that truly touches my heart. I receive calls from former clients who tell me about a sister, aunt, friend or neighbor whom they have helped because of what they have learned through the makeover program. That's what it's all about. With the knowledge comes the responsibility to share and touch other lives, thereby enriching them so they can be the full expression of what God intended them to be. May God bless you and keep you in vibrant health and give you the strength and courage to share the good news!

WHAT ABOUT THE EATING PLAN?

You should continue eating the same basic program but get creative. Use millet bread, tomatoes, rice, soy cheese and vegetables to make a small pizza. Roast vegetables with olive oil and serve with brown rice. Stir-fry, steam, roast or eat your foods raw. Eat only foods that are alive— foods that have not been stripped of nutrients. Eat often and eat early; do not eat late at night. Drink plenty of water and herb teas. If you ever stray from the basic program, just start over at the first 30-days section. You can always begin again, and you may have to! But you should be feeling so much better and in control of your eating that to stray from the basic plan almost seems unimaginable.

90 DAYS—SUCCESS!

It's time to chart your success! Now we are at the exciting part of your makeover. Here is the same immune response questionnaire you completed at 30 days. After completing the questionnaire now, compare it with your 30-day questionnaire. You should see remarkable differences and an elimination of most of the bothersome symptoms of lowered immune function. As you move forward from this 90-day mark, you will only grow stronger and more vibrant than ever before.

IMMUNE RESPONSE QUESTIONNAIRE

Instructions: Please circle the number that best describes the frequency or severity of your complaints. Leave the question blank if it does not apply to you.

0 = no symptoms   2 = moderate symptoms
1 = mild symptoms   3 = severe symptoms

Section A

1. Easily susceptible to infections	0	1	2	3
2. Frequently catch a cold or flu	0	1	2	3
3. Difficult to recuperate from a flu or cold	0	1	2	3
4. Chronic swollen lymph glands	0	1	2	3
5. Frequent sore throats	0	1	2	3
6. Cuts or bruises heal slowly	0	1	2	3
7. Hair grows slowly	0	1	2	3
8. Frequent ear infections	0	1	2	3
9. Cold sores or fever blisters	0	1	2	3
10. Chronic low-grade fever	0	1	2	3
11. Gums and/or nose bleeds easily	0	1	2	3
12. Experience frequent runny nose	0	1	2	3
13. Muscle aches and joint pain	0	1	2	3

Section B

1. Known chemical sensitivities	0	1	2	3
2. Known environmental and/or food allergies	0	1	2	3
3. Irritability/mood swings	0	1	2	3
4. Frequent headaches and/or migraines	0	1	2	3
5. Abnormal fatigue not helped by rest	0	1	2	3
6. Postnasal drip	0	1	2	3
7. Frequent sneezing attacks and/or hayfever	0	1	2	3
8. Weight fluctuations of four to five pounds in one day accompanied by puffiness in face/ankles/fingers	0	1	2	3
9. Chronic muscle aches and pains	0	1	2	3
10. Suffer from asthma/breathing difficulties	0	1	2	3
11. Eczema, hives or skin rashes	0	1	2	3
12. Suffer from depression or crying spells	0	1	2	3
13. Itchy eyes or nose	0	1	2	3
14. Chronic runny nose	0	1	2	3

15. Chronic stuffy nose	0	1	2	3
16. Dark circles under your eyes	0	1	2	3
17. Frequent urination or bedwetting	0	1	2	3
18. Swelling in joints	0	1	2	3
19. Mouth or throat itches	0	1	2	3
20. Chronic lymph gland swelling, especially in the throat area	0	1	2	3
21. Acne	0	1	2	3
22. Sweat for no apparent reason/hot flashes	0	1	2	3
23. Suffer from irritable bowel, spastic colon or colitis	0	1	2	3
24. Certain foods cause you to have a reaction (jitters, depression, ill feeling)	0	1	2	3
25. Strong cravings for certain foods	0	1	2	3
26. Pulse races after eating certain foods or for no apparent reason	0	1	2	3
27. Mucus in stool	0	1	2	3
28. Minor, chronic complaints that always reoccur	0	1	2	3
29. Feel best when you do not eat	0	1	2	3
30. Hyperactive	0	1	2	3
31. Abdominal pain after eating	0	1	2	3
32. Alternating diarrhea/constipation	0	1	2	3

Section C

1. Chronic fatigue, especially after eating	0	1	2	3
2. Depression	0	1	2	3
3. Recurrent digestive complaints	0	1	2	3
4. Rectal itching	0	1	2	3
5. Food and/or environmental allergies	0	1	2	3
6. Severe PMS	0	1	2	3
7. Feel "spacey"	0	1	2	3
8. Poor memory	0	1	2	3
9. Severe mood swings	0	1	2	3
10. Anxiety/nervousness	0	1	2	3
11. Recurrent fungal infections (athletes foot, ringworm, jock itch)	0	1	2	3
12. Extreme chemical sensitivity	0	1	2	3
13. Cannot tolerate perfumes or smoke	0	1	2	3
14. Coated or sore tongue	0	1	2	3

15. Prostatitis	0	1	2	3
16. Recurrent vaginal or urinary infections	0	1	2	3
17. Lightheadedness or feel drunk after minimal wine, beer or certain foods	0	1	2	3
18. Respiratory problems	0	1	2	3
19. Chronic skin rashes or acne	0	1	2	3
20. Loss of libido/impotence	0	1	2	3
21. Thrush	0	1	2	3
22. Headaches/migraines	0	1	2	3
23. Muscle and joint pains	0	1	2	3
24. Low blood sugar	0	1	2	3
25. History of frequent antibiotic use	0	1	2	3
26. Taking or have taken birth control pills	0	1	2	3
27. Crave sugar, breads or alcoholic beverages	0	1	2	3
28. Endometriosis and/or infertility	0	1	2	3
29. Above conditions get worse in moldy places like basements or damp climates	0	1	2	3
30. Above conditions get worse after eating or drinking items that contain yeast or sugar	0	1	2	3

Section D

1. Fatigue	0	1	2	3
2. Depression	0	1	2	3
3. Anxiety	0	1	2	3
4. High blood pressure	0	1	2	3
5. Increased susceptibility to infections	0	1	2	3
6. Headaches	0	1	2	3
7. Digestive problems (colic, nausea, pain)	0	1	2	3
8. Numbness/tingling/tremors	0	1	2	3
9. Skin problems (rashes, eczema, psoriasis)	0	1	2	3
10. Learning disabilities	0	1	2	3
11. Ringing in your ears	0	1	2	3
12. Muscle and joint pain	0	1	2	3
13. Allergies/asthma	0	1	2	3
14. Kidney and/or liver problems	0	1	2	3
15. Constipation	0	1	2	3
16. Memory problems	0	1	2	3
17. Anemia	0	1	2	3
18. Varied symptoms with no relief	0	1	2	3

TEN FUNCTIONAL FOODS THAT BUILD IMMUNITY

1. *Soy.* Twenty-five grams of soy protein a day may help lower cholesterol and reduce heart disease risk. Soy may also fight osteoporosis.
2. *Tomatoes.* Cooked, canned or ketchup are protective against prostate cancer when ten servings are consumed each week. They contain lycopene, which neutralizes harmful free radicals that can damage cells and trigger cancer.
3. *Oats.* Oats have been shown to reduce the risk of heart disease.
4. *Grapes.* Polyphenols or flavonoids in red grapes may lower the risk of stroke and heart disease.
5. *Tea.* One cup of green or black tea per day could cut the risk of heart attack by 44 percent.
6. *Citrus.* Fruits and juices contain high levels of vitamin C, potassium and folic acid.
7. *Fresh herbs.* Herbs are used to enhance the natural flavor of foods, thereby discouraging the overuse of butter and salt.
8. *Spinach.* One serving of spinach per week can protect against colon cancer, twice weekly to prevent cataracts. Its vitamin K content helps to build strong bones.
9. *Vegetables (cruciferous).* Eaten two to three times a week, these help prevent colon and lung cancer.
10. *Vegetables (beta carotene).* These are protective against heart diseases, stroke and some cancers.

IMMUNE-BOOSTING RECIPES

Now that you have learned how to eat for maximum immunity, it is time to add these delicious recipes to your eating plan. Notice how each recipe incorporates ingredients that boost immune function. *Bon appétit!*

Green Tea Chicken Salad

3 Tbsp. sesame oil
4 boneless, skinless chicken breasts
3 Tbsp. green tea leaves
½ c. cold spring water, plus ⅛ c. rice vinegar
½ tsp. Bragg's Liquid Aminos
⅛ tsp. stevia powder extract (or to taste)
¾ c. olive oil
½ c. slivered almonds (toasted)
1 can sliced water chestnuts, drained
1 head of romaine lettuce, torn into pieces

In a large skillet over medium heat, heat 2 tablespoons of sesame oil. Sauté chicken breasts until cooked, about 5 to 7 minutes on each side. Set them aside to cool. To make the dressing, steep green tea leaves in water and vinegar for at least 30 minutes. Strain and discard the tea leaves. Add the remaining sesame oil, Bragg's Liquid Aminos, stevia and olive oil and mix well. Tear the cooked chicken breasts into pieces. Combine with toasted slivered almonds, water chestnuts and romaine lettuce. Add dressing and serve immediately. Serves 4.

You may want to have a glass of iced green tea sweetened with stevia extract along with this wonderful salad.

Immune-Boosting Antipasto Salad

½ head cauliflower, separated into bite-sized pieces
2 large carrots, cut into 2-in. match sticks
1 each large red, yellow and green bell peppers, cut into ½-in. strips
½ lb. Shiitake mushrooms (small, otherwise halve them)
1 package frozen artichoke hearts
⅓ c. olive oil
½ c. apple cider vinegar
3 Tbsp. Dijon mustard
1 garlic clove, minced
1 tsp. oregano
1 tsp. sea salt
½ tsp. black pepper
1 bunch scallions (6 to 8), coarsely chopped
2 c. cubed cooked chicken or turkey (about ½ lb.)

Place the cauliflower, carrots, bell peppers and mushrooms in a large steamer; steam until tender, about 6 minutes. Add the artichokes for the last 3 or 4 minutes of steaming to thaw them. Meanwhile, in a small bowl or measuring cup, combine the oil, vinegar, mustard, garlic, oregano, sea salt and black pepper. Transfer the steamed vegetables to a large bowl and top with dressing. Add the scallions and meat to the vegetables; toss to coat well. Set aside for 3 hours in the refrigerator. Remove from the refrigerator approximately 30 minutes before serving to allow it to come to room temperature. This will keep for up to 3 days in refrigerator, stirring occasionally. Serves 4.

FRUIT AND YOGURT PARFAITS

¼ c. slivered almonds
¼ c. flaked coconut
¼ c. raisins
2 medium peaches, thinly sliced
2 medium plums, thinly sliced
2 c. strawberries, halved
½ c. plain yogurt
½ tsp. vanilla extract
2 Tbsp. honey or 1 tsp. stevia extract

In a small ungreased skillet, toast the almonds and coconut over medium heat until coconut is golden, about 6 minutes. Set aside to cool slightly, then stir in the raisins. Combine peaches, plums and strawberries in a medium bowl. In a separate small bowl, stir together the yogurt, honey (or stevia) and vanilla. Layer the fruit and yogurt mixture in 4 parfait or other tall glasses, adding 1 tablespoon of the coconut mixture to each glass when it is half filled. Top the parfaits with the remaining coconut mixture. Makes 4 parfaits.

PASTA IMMUNIVERA

1 lb. fresh asparagus
2 c. fresh broccoli flowerets
1 medium onion
1 large clove garlic, chopped
1 Tbsp. olive oil
1 large carrot, scraped and diagonally sliced
1 each medium red and yellow pepper, coarsely chopped

1 c. rice milk
1 tsp. arrowroot powder
½ c. chicken broth
3 green onions, chopped
2 Tbsp. chopped fresh basil (or 2 tsp. dried whole basil)
½ tsp. sea salt
8 oz. uncooked spinach pasta
½ lb. Shiitake mushrooms, sliced
1 c. shredded rice cheese
¼ tsp. freshly ground pepper

Snap off tough ends of asparagus. Remove scales with a vegetable peeler or knife, if desired. Cut asparagus diagonally into 1½-inch pieces. Place asparagus pieces and broccoli flowerets in a vegetable steamer over boiling water; cover and steam 6 to 8 minutes or until vegetables are crisp tender. Remove from heat and set aside. Sauté onion and garlic in oil in a large skillet until tender. Add carrot and chopped peppers to onion mixture; sauté until crisp tender. Remove from heat and drain. Combine rice milk, arrowroot powder, broth, green onions, basil and sea salt in a medium skillet. Cook over medium-high heat for 5 minutes, stirring occasionally. Cook spinach pasta according to package directions. Drain well; place in a large serving bowl. Add reserved vegetables, rice milk mixture and sliced mushrooms; toss gently. Sprinkle with rice cheese and pepper; toss gently. Serve immediately. Serves 4.

LAYERED FRUIT SALAD

1 lb. grapes
2 bananas
1 can (16 oz.) or 4 fresh peaches, sliced
1 pint fresh raspberries
2 oranges
3 kiwis
Juice from 2 additional oranges
1 tsp. powdered stevia extract

Rinse grapes. Cut in half and remove seeds. Place in bottom of a glass serving bowl. Peel and slice bananas; place over grapes. Drain peaches well and cut into smaller pieces; distribute on top of bananas. Carefully rinse raspberries. Sprinkle on top of bananas. Peel oranges, removing the white skin. Slice and cut into smaller pieces. Place on top of raspberries. Peel and slice kiwis. Garnish salad. Pour orange juice over top of salad and sprinkle with stevia if desired. Keep salad refrigerated until ready to serve. Serves 4.

BARBECUE-ROASTED TURKEY BREAST

1 medium onion, coarsely chopped
⅔ c. ketchup
2 Tbsp. tomato paste
2 Tbsp. Bragg's Liquid Aminos
2 Tbsp. olive oil
2 Tbsp. apple cider vinegar
1 Tbsp. Worcestershire sauce
½ tsp. stevia powder extract
2 tsp. dry mustard
1 boneless turkey breast half (about 3.5 lbs.)

Preheat oven to 425 degrees. Line a roasting pan with foil. Combine all ingredients except turkey in a small saucepan. Bring to a boil over medium-high heat, stirring until well blended. Remove the pan from the heat and set aside. Place the turkey breast on the prepared roasting pan. Brush the turkey with ¼ of the barbecue sauce. Roast the turkey for 15 minutes. Reduce the oven temperature to 325 degrees. Brush the turkey with most of the remaining sauce; roast, basting periodically, until the turkey registers 170 degrees on a meat thermometer, about 1 hour and 45 minutes. Let the turkey stand for 5 to 10 minutes before slicing and serving. Serve any leftover basting sauce on the side. Serve with a vegetable or a side of brown rice. Serves 4.

BELL PEPPERS STUFFED WITH CORN, BEANS AND RICE

1½ c. low-sodium chicken broth
2 plum tomatoes or 2 whole canned tomatoes, well
  drained and coarsely chopped
1 small onion, coarsely chopped
¼ c. fresh basil leaves, minced
3 cloves garlic, minced or crushed
2 Tbsp. lemon juice
3 tsp. grated lemon peel
1 tsp. oregano
¼ tsp. black pepper

½ c. corn
¾ c. brown rice (raw)
4 large bell peppers (yellow and red)
1 c. black canned beans, rinsed and drained
3 Tbsp. rice cheese, shredded

In a medium saucepan, bring the chicken broth to a boil over medium-high heat. Add the tomatoes, onion, basil leaves, garlic, lemon juice, lemon peel, oregano, black pepper, corn and rice. Return to a boil, and then reduce heat to low; cover and simmer until the rice is tender and has absorbed all the liquid, about 20 minutes. Preheat oven to 350 degrees. Meanwhile, cut an opening in the tops of the bell peppers and remove the stems, seeds and ribs, leaving the rest of the pepper intact. Stand peppers upright in a baking dish. Stir the black beans into the cooked rice. Dividing evenly, stuff the peppers with the rice mixture. Top with shredded rice cheese. Bake 15 minutes, or until the cheese is golden. Serves 4.

BROILED FISH STEAKS WITH TOMATO-BELL PEPPER RELISH

4 medium plum tomatoes or 1 can (14 oz.) whole tomatoes,
    well drained, coarsely chopped
1 small red bell pepper
3 scallions
¼ c. fresh basil leaves
2 Tbsp. olive oil
2 Tbsp. apple cider vinegar
½ tsp. black pepper
¼ tsp. sea salt
4 tuna, cod or halibut steaks, about ¾-in. thick

Preheat the broiler. Line a broiler pan with foil and lightly grease the foil. In a food processor, coarsely chop the bell pepper, scallions and basil. Transfer the vegetable mixture to a bowl. Stir in the chopped tomatoes, olive oil, vinegar, black pepper and sea salt; stir well. Place the fish steaks on the prepared broiler pan. Strain the excess liquid from the tomato-bell pepper relish into a small bowl. Brush the fish with some of the liquid and broil 4 inches from the heat for 4 minutes. Turn the fish over and brush with more of the liquid; broil until the fish flakes when tested with a fork, about 4 minutes longer. Serve the steaks topped with the tomato-bell pepper relish. Serves 4.

179

A+ CURRIED CARROT SOUP

6 medium carrots, peeled
1 large sweet potato
1 bunch scallions (6 to 8)
2 Tbsp. unsalted butter
2 cloves garlic, minced
3 c. fat-free chicken broth
3 Tbsp. curry powder
$\frac{1}{4}$ tsp. pepper
$\frac{1}{2}$ c. plain yogurt

Cut the carrots into large pieces. Cut the sweet potato into large chunks. Coarsely chop the scallions, keeping the white and green portions separate from the dark green tops. In a large saucepan, warm the butter over medium-high heat until it is melted. Add the scallion whites and garlic; cook until the scallions are translucent, about 3 minutes. Add the carrots, sweet potato, chicken broth, curry powder and pepper; cover and bring to a boil over medium-high heat. Reduce the heat to low, and simmer until the carrots and sweet potato are tender, about 20 minutes. With a slotted spoon, transfer the solids to a food processor or blender and puree. Return the puree to the broth in the pan and stir to blend. Serve topped with a dollop of yogurt and a sprinkling of scallion greens. Serves 2.

TURKEY SCALOPPINI WITH BELL PEPPERS AND SHIITAKE MUSHROOMS

2 Tbsp. arrowroot powder
$\frac{3}{4}$ tsp. oregano
$\frac{1}{2}$ tsp. sea salt
$\frac{1}{4}$ tsp. black pepper
4 turkey cutlets
1 Tbsp. olive oil
$\frac{1}{4}$ lb. shiitake mushrooms
1 medium red bell pepper
$\frac{1}{2}$ c. fat-free chicken broth
1 medium yellow bell pepper
3 Tbsp. fresh parsley

In a plastic or paper bag combine the arrowroot powder, $\frac{1}{2}$ teaspoon of oregano, the sea salt and black pepper. Add turkey cutlets, and lightly dredge them in the seasoned arrowroot mixture. In a large skillet, preferably nonstick, warm the olive oil over medium-high heat until hot, but not smoking. Add the turkey and cook until light golden on both sides, 3 to 4 minutes per side. Meanwhile, slice the mushrooms, ¼ inch thick. Cut the peppers into strips ¼ inch wide. Remove the turkey from the skillet, and cover loosely to keep warm. Add the bell peppers, shiitake mushrooms, chicken broth and remaining ¼ teaspoon oregano to the skillet. Reduce heat to medium; cover and simmer for 3 minutes. Return the turkey to the pan. Increase the heat to medium-high; cover and cook until the turkey is heated through, about 2 minutes. Serve the turkey with the vegetables and steamed brown rice with pan juices paired on top. Sprinkle with fresh parsley. Serves 4.

PARSLEY SPREAD

Parsley is a diuretic that purifies the blood and accelerates the excretion of toxins. Eaten regularly, it reduces heart rate and lowers blood pressure. Chew on parsley leaves after dinner to keep your breath fresh. Parsley ranks higher than most vegetables in histidine, an amino acid that inhibits tumors. Keep your parsley fresh by sprinkling it with water, then wrapping it in a paper towel and refrigerating it in a plastic bag.

2 bunches parsley
2 shallots
½ c. plain yogurt
1 c. silken tofu
2 Tbsp. lemon juice
2 scallions
4 large tomatoes
Pinch salt
Pinch cayenne pepper

Wash parsley in cold water and strip the leaves from the stalks. Coarsely chop the parsley. Then peel and dice the shallots. Mix together the yogurt, tofu, lemon juice, parsley and diced shallots. Peel the scallions and cut into thin rings. Dice two tomatoes, season with salt and cayenne pepper to taste, and mix with the scallions. Cut the remaining two tomatoes into ½-inch slices. Cover them with the parsley spread and top with the tomato-scallion mixture.

TEST YOUR KNOWLEDGE

Now it's time to show me what you have learned. Remember, with knowledge comes responsibility to share and help others. Where have we heard this before? "To whom much is given, from him much will be required" (Luke 12:48, NKJV).

The following exercise will show you where you need to study a little more when it comes to building optimal immune health. I have created a client for you to work with—Miserable Mabel. What body-balancing recommendations would you make for her?

Client History
Name: Miserable Mabel
Age: 50

Check all symptoms that apply:

Gastrointestinal
- ☑ Digestive complaints
- ☑ Stomach pain
- ❏ Ulcers
- ☑ Frequent heartburn
- ☑ Frequent constipation
- ❏ Frequent diarrhea
- ❏ Irritable bowel
- ❏ Hemorrhoids
- ❏ Frequent vomiting
- ❏ Colitis
- ☑ Gallbladder trouble
- ☑ Frequent burping/belching

Immune response
- ☑ Frequently sick
- ☑ Frequent swollen glands/sore throats
- ❏ Depression and/or anxiety

- ☑ Achy joints/muscle pain
- ☑ Headaches/Migraines
- ☑ Recurrent digestive complaints
- ❑ Chronic fatigue
- ❑ Food allergies
- ❑ Eczema or hives
- ❑ Allergies

Structural/neurological

- ☑ Headaches
- ☑ Muscle cramps/spasms
- ☑ Neck pain
- ❑ Jaw pain
- ❑ Dizziness
- ☑ Back pain
- ❑ Shoulder/elbow/wrist pain
- ❑ Numbness/tingling
- ❑ Tremors in hands or feet
- ☑ Knee pain/hip pain
- ❑ Joint pain or loss of function
- ☑ Osteoporosis or osteomalacia
- ❑ Current bone fracture or injury
- ❑ Tendonitis/bursitis

Cardiovascular

- ☑ Irregular heartbeat
- ☑ Heart murmur/ palpitations
- ☑ High or low blood pressure
- ❑ Chest pain
- ❑ Previous heart trouble
- ❑ Poor circulation
- ❑ Previous heart surgery
- ❑ Varicose or spider veins
- ❑ Hands and feet cold all the time
- ☑ High cholesterol

Respiratory

- ☑ Chronic cough
- ❑ Asthma
- ❑ Emphysema

☑ Recurrent head colds
☑ Recurrent sinus infections
❑ Recurrent bronchitis
☑ Smoker

Genito-urinary

❑ Too frequent urination
❑ Blood in urine
☑ Recurrent kidney or bladder infections
❑ Kidney stones
❑ Bedwetting
❑ Inability to control bladder

Endocrine glandular

❑ Cold hands and feet
❑ Low blood pressure
☑ Weight problems
☑ Thyroid problems
❑ Diabetes
❑ Irritable if meals are missed
☑ Anxiety/nervousness/irritability
❑ Dizzy upon standing too quickly
☑ Weak and shaky
❑ Hyperactive behavior
☑ Depression
❑ Very susceptible to infections
❑ Frequent headaches
☑ Digestive complaints
❑ Yeast infections
❑ Menstrual irregularity
❑ Cramping
❑ Mood swings/depression
❑ Infertility
❑ Frequent miscarriages
☑ Hot flashes
❑ Taking hormone medication
❑ Taking birth control pills
☑ Lumps in breast
❑ Uterine cysts/ovarian cysts
☑ Endometriosis

Miscellaneous
- ☑ Difficulty sleeping
- ☑ Restless, uneasy sleep
- ❑ Edema

List any symptoms or unusual conditions you feel are important:

1. I feel miserable! Sincerely, Mabel

What do you recommend for Mabel?

Gastrointestinal	Structural/neurological
1. _____	1. _____
2. _____	2. _____
3. _____	3. _____
4. _____	4. _____
5. _____	5. _____
6. _____	6. _____

Immune response	Cardiovascular
1. _____	1. _____
2. _____	2. _____
3. _____	3. _____
4. _____	4. _____
5. _____	5. _____
6. _____	6. _____

Respiratory	Genito-urinary
1. _____	1. _____
2. _____	2. _____
3. _____	3. _____
4. _____	4. _____
5. _____	5. _____
6. _____	6. _____
7. _____	7. _____

Endocrine Glandular	*Miscellaneous*
1. _____	1. _____
2. _____	2. _____
3. _____	3. _____
4. _____	4. _____
5. _____	5. _____

RATE YOUR IMMUNE-BOOSTING SKILLS

The following summaries are recommendations that I would make for Mabel. Compare your recommendations with those listed below.

Gastrointestinal

First, Mabel needs to detoxify her body and begin the 90-Day Immune System Makeover eating plan. She also needs to supplement her system with plant digestive enzymes. I recommend Lypo from Enzymedica for her because she has high cholesterol and is overweight. In addition, she needs to add probiotics to improve her intestinal health. Kyo-Green or liquid chlorophyll is another tool she will need to add for digestive health. Mabel also needs to undertake a liver/gallbladder flush to eliminate small stones and enhance the function of both organs. Mabel needs to add fiber to her diet either from dietary sources or by supplementation. Chamomile tea is a good nighttime treat.

Dr. Janet's recommendations

1. Detoxify
2. Lypo
3. Kyo-Green
4. Probiotic/acidophilus
5. Liver flush
6. Add fiber to diet/chamomile tea

Immune response

Since Mabel checked frequently sick with frequent swollen glands, I recommend astragalus to boost her immunity along with the power mushroom reishi, which will also help to lower her cholesterol. Echinachea will boost her white cell count to help her immune system fight infection, but not for long term use. For her headaches, achy joints and muscle pain, I recommend CalMax Pain, Back and Stress Powder to tackle this problem. I also recommend a soothing warm bath with sea salt and baking soda with lavender essential oil added for stress relief.

Dr. Janet's recommendations
1. Astragalus
2. Reishi
3. Echinachea
4. CalMax
5. Bath with lavender oil

Structural/neurological

Mabel is very uncomfortable with headaches, muscle cramps, neck pain, back pain, knee pain, hip pain and osteoporosis. I recommend CalMax twice daily, morning and night, and Dr. Janet's Glucosamine Cream applied topically to just about every inch of her body (neck, back, knees and hip). Essential fatty acids are needed as well as antioxidants to help quench excessive free radicals that are associated with pain syndromes. Again, therapeutic baths will help Mabel tremendously. In addition, Dr. Janet's Progesterone Cream will help her osteoporosis.

Dr. Janet's recommendations
1. CalMax
2. Essential fatty acids
3. Dr. Janet's Glucosamine Cream
4. Therapeutic warm bath
5. Dr. Janet's Progesterone Cream
6. Antioxidants

Cardiovascular

CalMax will help Mabel's irregular heartbeat, palpitations and high blood pressure. It may be hard at first, but Mabel needs to get moving with some form of exercise. In addition, Mabel needs to take coenzyme Q_{10}, 90 milligrams daily, for cardiovascular health along with lecithin to help her body emulsify fats and lower cholesterol. Red yeast rice also helps, as does L-carnitine, Kyolic Garlic Extract and guggul, in the battle against high cholesterol levels. All of the abovementioned supplements will help the entire cardiovascular system.

Dr. Janet's recommendations
1. CalMax
2. Coenzyme Q_{10}
3. Exercise
4. Kyolic Garlic Extract
5. Red yeast rice
6. Guggul

Respiratory

Since Mabel has recurrent sinus infections and head colds, I recommend astragalus, reishi mushroom and short-term echinachea use. In addition, she should eliminate wheat and dairy completely from her diet and switch to millet-grain bread and soy or rice milk. This will cut down on her mucous production. And last but not least, Mabel needs to stop smoking.

Dr. Janet's recommendations
1. Astragalus
2. Reishi mushrooms
3. Echinachea
4. Eliminate wheat and dairy
5. Millet bread and rice or soy milk
6. Stop smoking

Genito-urinary
Mabel needs to take cranberry capsules to get her bladder acidified in order to control bacterial growth. Antioxidants, biotic silver, probiotics and Kyo-Green or chlorophyll each day will also help. She needs to drink pure water and stay away from sugary-sweet juices and colas.

Dr. Janet's recommendations
1. Cranberry capsules
2. Biotic silver
3. Antioxidants
4. Probiotics
5. Kyo-Green
6. More purified water
7. Avoid sugary beverages

Endocrine glandular
Mabel has checked anxiety, nervousness, irritability and depression. I recommend that she give GABA a try. She should get a formula that contains GABA, inositol and niacinamide for extra relaxation benefits. She also

complains of hot flashes, endometriosis and lumps in her breast. She has the indications of estrogen dominance. I recommend Dr. Janet's Natural Progesterone Cream to balance the ratio of estrogen to progesterone; this will help her breast lumps, discourage overgrowth of endo-metrium and as an added bonus, enhance her thyroid activity. This in turn will help her lose weight. Of course, exercise and the immune-eating plan will also contribute to weight loss. Kyo-Green will also help thyroid function.

Dr. Janet's recommendations
1. GABA
2. Progesterone cream
3. Kyo-Green

Miscellaneous
Mabel needs a good night's sleep. CalMax will come to her rescue. I recommend that she add CalMax powder to a cup of hot chamomile tea. If she needs additional help, she may try a capsule of valerian root or a GABA capsule before bed. She should also eliminate caffeine.

Dr. Janet's recommendations
1. CalMax
2. Chamomile tea
3. Valerian
4. GABA
5. Eliminate caffeine

MEDICINE IN THE MILLENNIUM

As I was writing this book, a very timely medical sympo-sium was held in my hometown, "Medicine in the Millennium." I am sure that you will be interested in the very latest information that was shared. After reading it, I am sure that you will agree and even be more strongly convinced that only by boosting your immune function, managing stress and staying in the Word of God can you achieve and maintain vibrant health!

Dr. Richard Duma, director of infectious disease at Halifax Medical Center and a speaker at the symposium stated that "every infectious disease has been on the increase in the last twenty years, not a decrease despite all the antibiotics we have." Even as medical science advances, bacteria are becoming increasingly resistant to antibiotics, new diseases crop up every year, and old diseases that had at one time become scarce are becoming prevalent once again.

In the last fifty years, a long and troubling list of new viruses, bacteria and diseases has emerged: HIV, AIDS, Ebola, *hantavirus, E. coli, cryptosporidiosis,* Legionnaire's disease and *pfiesteriosis.* Amoebae-laden lakes are becoming prevalent. Diseases once in decline are making a comeback, including tuberculosis, diphtheria and trench fever. Why is this occurring? It is believed to be caused by our increasingly mobile society, which makes the transport of viruses from one hemisphere to another possible, coupled with a growing population sprawling into unpopulated regions and an international food trade that is not subject to America's quality controls.

A generation ago, a leading expert predicted that the introduction of penicillin would soon eradicate infectious disease as a threat to public health. Today's physicians warn that emerging diseases should not be taken lightly. They are not considered somebody else's problem. We have become a global family. Take last year's outback of West Nile encephalitis in New York City! Health officials elsewhere are concerned, including my home state of Florida, because the virus is caused by birds—and birds migrate.

Antibiotics are becoming less effective in killing bacteria. Pneumonia and meningitis are now becoming resistant to penicillin, and a population of resistant bacteria is thriving. According to Dr. Duma, we will never solve the resistant problem, and new antibiotics alone are not the answer. In conclusion, coupled with the emergence of new diseases and the lessening effectiveness of the world's current antibiotics, the twenty-first century will be the most challenging one of epidemiologists.

This is why boosting our immunity is crucial.

NEWS FLASH!

Research at the University of Illinois has discovered that 80 percent of the bacteria in human colons contain genes allowing for the bacteria to become antibiotic resistant. Thirty years ago, less than 33 percent of these bacteria were found to contain these genes.

Researcher Abigail Salyers, Ph.D., professor of microbiology, presented her findings at the Sixth Annual Midwest Microbial Pathogens Meeting in Milwaukee, Wisconsin, in September of 1999. She pointed out that the presence of this bacteria should be a wake-up call to the medical community. "Resistant bacteria are now entering our food supply and might donate their resistance genes to human bacteria," said Dr. Salyers. "I am not saying that the agricultural use of antibiotics is causing the problem, just that it is a possible factor. So let's find out." Other researchers believe that giving antibiotics to cows, chickens, pigs and other food sources has contributed in a big way to the bacteria that cannot be killed by antibiotics.

This only confirms that you must keep your immune system in tiptop shape by eating plenty of fruits and vegetables, taking antioxidants, getting enough sleep, drinking plenty of pure water and eliminating fast foods, junk foods and everything that takes away from optimal body performance.

IMMUNE-BOOSTING FOODS

In my continuing journey for optimal immune health, I am always updating my list of immune-boosting foods, supplements, herbs, vitamins and minerals. God has provided us with everything we need, not only in our physical bodies but also in nature. I want to share with you some of my favorite immune system fortifiers and boosters that my clients have come to love as well. They truly make a difference. Just try any one of the following gifts from God's garden, and experience a higher level of health. In our generation, we are learning more and more about the health-building properties of specific foods and supplements. Science is finally finding out that our foods are truly "the best medicine" for our body. Technology has advanced so much in our generation. Genetic research into plant metabolism has made possible powerful neutraceuticals for therapeutic use.

Let's begin with one of my favorites—royal jelly. First let me tell you what it is. It's called royal jelly because it is fed exclusively to the queen bee by the nurse-worker bees. It is a milky secretion produced from the head glands of the nurse-worker bees. When the queen is fed the royal jelly, she outlives the other bees by many years. Royal jelly is brimming with amino acids, vitamins and minerals. It is a natural immune system builder, especially nourishing to the adrenal glands. Remember, these glands are very important for a multitude of bodily functions. In addition, it is a natural antibiotic, antibacterial and antiviral agent. It helps to combat stress and promotes longevity.

Next on my list is garlic. Often called Russian penicillin, garlic is a proven blood cleanser, cancer fighter and natural antibiotic. In the times of Moses, garlic was readily used as an anticoagulant, antiseptic, anti-inflammatory agent and a tumor fighter. Researchers at Loma Linda University in California have shown the Kyolic Garlic from Wakunaga reduces LDL levels in the blood while increasing beneficial HDL. Other studies have shown that garlic can lower your blood cholesterol level dramatically in 60 days.

Astragalus is probably a new supplement for you, but the truth is that it has been used for centuries as a powerful immune enhancer and body tonic. I have used astragalus on and off for years during times when I felt that my immune response needed boosting. This is another all-time favorite of my clients. In addition to immune boosting, it is antiviral, can help lower blood pressure, can improve circulation and can act as a natural diuretic.

Now we are going to get a little exotic—mushrooms. Not just any mushroom, but a wonderful, powerful immune-boosting mushroom—reishi. Research in China and the United States backs up reishi's health-restoring properties. Studies are being conducted on reishi's possible benefit on chronic fatigue syndrome, asthma, arthritis and cancer. The reason it is so effective is that it contains properties that reduces cholesterol, normalizes blood pressure, fights cancer and prevents blood platelets from clumping. In addition, it relaxes the body by helping to control the release of adrenaline. The next power mushroom is maitake. It is grown in northeastern Japan and is the most potent immune stimulator of all of the power mushrooms. There are reports that maitake can actually cause tumors to shrink. Maitake has also proven itself valuable for people with Epstein-Barr virus, high blood pressure and diabetes. Much research into AIDS is now being undertaken concerning maitake's effect on HIV.

Maitake, reishi, astragalus, royal jelly, and garlic are all available at your local health food stores.

THE NEW CANCER FIGHTER—IP 6

An exciting discovery has been made. An important component of cereals and legumes may be the active ingredient in fiber that is anticarcinogenic. It's called IP6. Currently, there are a growing number of studies that support the cancer-fighting properties of this wonderful substance. IP6 may prove to be the best new medicine for the new millennium.

The University of Maryland in Baltimore studied whether a high-fiber diet reduced the amount of tumor cells in rats. They divided rats into five groups and fed them a diet consisting of 0 percent, 5 percent, 10 percent or 20 percent of Kellogg's All Bran Cereal; a fifth group received 0.4 percent IP6 in their drinking water, which is an amount equal to 20 percent bran. After twenty-nine weeks, they found that in the 5 to 20 percent bran cereal groups, tumor incidence decreased 11 to 17 percent. Interestingly enough, the rats that ate the least amount of bran had a lower tumor incidence than the group that are the most bran. The researchers concluded that we do not have to fill ourselves with bran in order to reap the benefits. What would happen if we drank the IP6? The rats that were given the IP6 in their water had an even lower incidence of tumor formation. It was exciting to discover that drinking the IP6 seemed to work twice as well as eating high-bran foods. Scientists have also discovered that cancer cells can revert back to normal in the presence of IP6. It should be noted that most of this research has been performed on animals. More human trials need to be done in order to gain more support from the medical community.

One of the nations experts in IP6, Abulkalam Shamsuddin, M.D., has authored a book entitled *IP6— Nature's Revolutionary Cancer Fighter,* and he states that the quality of fiber you eat is more important than the quantity. He gives the example of Finnish and Danish populations. Danes eat twice as much fiber as the Finns, yet Danes have twice the amount of cancer as the Finns. Shamsuddin states that this is because Finns eat a lot of porridge, which is rich in IP6, while Danes eat a lot of fiber that does not contain IP6. Corn contains the highest concentration of IP6, followed by sesame, wheat and rice respectively. IP6 is available in pill or powder form in health food stores across the country. There are no known side effects or toxicity. Supplemental IP6 is recommended because not all IP6 can be absorbed from foods.

As of this date, the recommended dosage for prevention is 1 to 2 grams per day. Those with a family risk of cancer or who have a high-risk lifestyle, such as smoking and exposure to chemicals and pesticides, should take 4 grams daily. If you are battling cancer, the recommended dose is 8 grams daily. Expect to hear more about IP6 in the next year. Much excitement has been generated in the scientific research area concerning this cancer fighter that is also an antioxidant, as well as an effective treatment for high cholesterol and kidney stones. The American Cancer Society has requested information on IP6 and is currently evaluating the research that has been done. I expect to see IP6 in the protocol for cancer patients within the next five years.

Many people have already begun to take IP6 because of its safety. If you wish to incorporate IP6 into your immune-boosting plan, you may do so. If you are in doubt, seek the guidance of your health care professional so they may help you plan either a preventative or treatment for cancer protocol that will include IP6.

Learning to Adapt With Adaptogens

In my continuing search for immune enhancement, I often come across remarkable substances that naturally support immune function. I am pleased to inform you of an herb from China that is virtually unknown in America. But not for long. I believe that very shortly our country will be buzzing about this newcomer called *Jiaogulan*, pronounced "je-ow-goo-lan." Jiaogulan is an adaptogenic herb that can help protect the body from the stresses of cancer therapy. In addition, taking adaptogenic herbs, like Jiaogulan, can result in normalized blood pressure, blood lipids, blood sugar and blood oxygen levels. This means that they are used in cases of hypertension, hyperlipidemia, diabetes and altitude sickness. Adaptogens can help enhance sports performance, mental focus and vitality. You can imagine how intrigued I was to learn that this ancient herb falls under the same category as ginseng. The entire world knows the benefit of ginseng. You can even purchase it at your local 7-Eleven or gas station these days. That's how mainstream America it has become. Move over, ginseng, because various Chinese clinical trials have shown that Jiaogulan is safe and has both chemical constituents and herbal properties comparable to ginseng. Others feel that it may even be superior to ginseng because it has a broader range of benefits!

In an earlier section, I told you about the importance of antioxidants in our battle against free-radical damage. You will be happy to learn that Jiaogulan is not only an adaptogen but an antioxidant as well. For those of you who do not know exactly what an adaptogen is, it very simply is a substance that enhances immunity, has a normalizing action on various bodily functions and helps to bring about "homeostasis" or equilibrium to the body.

We mentioned the importance of stress management by exercising, nutrition, relaxation, prayer and dietary supplement in the section of stress and immunity. We know that constant unrelenting stress will gradually weaken even the healthiest of persons who do not take the steps needed to improve the balance in their lives. This is where Jiaogulan can be a true blessing. By increasing adaptogenic and antioxidant supplementation, we can help support the body's defenses against stress. Without antioxidant and adaptogenic protection, our bodies will likely be adversely affected by stress-related illness and accelerated aging. Adaptogenic herbs such as Jiaogulan help our bodies to adapt and counteract the effects of stress. In addition, they help to strengthen our immune defense, nourishing those very important adrenal glands while boosting the body's energy.

In individuals who are battling stress, an adaptogenic herb like Jiaogulan will both mentally and physically help the body withstand and counteract the effects of excessive stress. In healthy individuals, Jiaogulan can enhance their general health and performance. I have had the pleasure of having many phone conversations with Michael Blumert, owner of Golden Mountain Herb Products, Inc. in Badger, California. His company works in conjunction with Guryang Medical College, where a number of clinical studies on Jiaogulan were done. They are a manufacturer of Jiaogulan-based products distributed directly to customers and health food stores across the country. It was Michael who first told me about Jiaogulan and its therapeutic health enriching benefits.

In 1976, a Japanese researcher, looking for a sugar alternative, studied a perennial weed known for its sweetness. He discovered this herb had qualities very similar to ginseng, even though unrelated as a plant. This one event sparked years of scientific research on the herb Jiaogulan, revealing it to be a very powerful adaptogenic and antioxidant herb with many therapeutic qualities. Since this herb is a new one for most of my readers, I am going to delve deeply into its benefit to the immune system. Jiaogulan has been shown in scientific studies to have the following therapeutic qualities:

- Antioxidant
- Adaptogen
- Enhances cardiovascular function

- Lowers high blood pressure
- Lowers cholesterol
- Strengthens immunity
- Inhibits cancer
- Prevents heart attack and stroke
- Strengthens our body's resistance.

The following dosages of Jiaogulan are based upon medical research studies and those recommended on commercial products sold in China:

- For antioxidant protection, 20 mg., three times daily
- An adaptogen, 20 mg. three times a day
- For improved and enhanced cardiovascular function, 20 mg. two or three times daily
- General illness prevention, 20 mg. two or three times daily
- To lower blood pressure–preventative dose, 20 mg. two or three times daily; therapeutic, 60 mg. two or three times daily
- Lowering cholesterol–preventative, 20 mg. two or three times daily; therapeutic, 60 mg. three times daily
- Protection against heart attack and stroke by inhibiting platelet aggregation–preventative, 20 mg. one or two times daily; therapeutic, 60 mg. three times daily
- Enhancing resistance by boosting white cell formation, therapeutic during radiation and chemotherapy, 60 mg. three times daily
- To strengthen immunity, 60 mg. two or three times daily

- Cancer prevention, 20 mg. two times daily; therapeutic, 60 mg. three times daily;
- Diabetes, liver disorders, bronchitis, 20 mg. three times daily.

FREQUENTLY ASKED QUESTIONS ABOUT JIAOGULAN

1. **Is Jiaogulan addicting?** No, not at all. It is a system balancer. It calms the brain when it is irritated and excites it when it is depressed, but it is neither a central nervous system stimulant nor a sedative.
2. **What effect does Jiaogulan have on my blood pressure?** It has a regulating effect. It helps to lower high blood pressure and raise low blood pressure. If your blood pressure is within normal limits, it does not affect your blood pressure at all.
3. **How can Jiaogulan help to relieve stress?** Through adjusting the balance of the central nervous system, which includes the brain, the sympathetic and parasympathetic nervous systems, and toning the endocrine system, it maintains and normalizes the functional equilibrium between the organs and the stability of the organism, thereby relieving stress.
4. **I already take antioxidants. Why should I take Jiaogulan?** Jiaogulan induces the body's own production of SOD, which is a strong, natural free-radical scavenger, thus protecting cells from free radical damage. It will also act in symphony or synergy with other antioxidants, such as vitamins A, C, E and selenium to increase the antioxidant effect.
5. **Is Jiaogulan beneficial for menopause?** Yes, because it adjusts the neuro-endocrine regulation of the genital system as well as balances the brain, the activity of the central nervous system, parasympathetic and sympathetic nervous systems, thus relieving menopausal symptoms.

If you want to experience the benefits of Jiaogulan for yourself, I have included the ordering information at the back of the book.

LOVABLE LECITHIN
BENEFITS BRAIN AND BODY

One of the easiest ways to enhance the health of your brain, nervous system, cardiovascular system, liver and other vital parts of your body is to supplement your body with lecithin. It has been said that lecithin does more to improve and preserve your health than any other nutrient.

Lecithin is found in virtually every cell of our body and is most concentrated in our liver, kidneys and brain. I have recommended lecithin to people with high blood lipids and high total cholesterol since lecithin helps to dissolve fats and cholesterol by acting as an emulsifier. I can tell you they have gotten great results and now make it a part of their daily protocol. Do you need to supplement your body with a daily dose of lecithin? You be the judge. The following information will help you make a quick decision about this nutrient.

Scientific studies show that we can repress or minimize age-related changes in our brain such as memory loss associated with aging by long-term use of a lecithin supplement. This is very exciting for older persons and those who battle higher than normal cholesterol. Dietary sources of lecithin in the amounts needed to be therapeutic and effective are very few. That's why I recommend supplementation with lecithin granules. Are you convinced yet? If not, read on. In your liver, lecithin metabolizes clogging fat, thereby reducing the chance of liver degeneration. In your bloodstream, as mentioned earlier, lecithin prevents cholesterol fats from accumulating on the walls of your arteries and can possibly help to dissolve any deposits that may already be there. Lecithin helps the absorption of vitamins and other nutrients in your intestinal tract. In addition, lecithin benefits the nervous system, skin and distribution of body fat. I personally take lecithin for the fat emulsifying and brain tonic properties.

Also, there is a family history of high cholesterol and heart disease in my family, so I make sure to take my lecithin daily. Two teaspoons daily may be added to food or juice. Lecithin is derived from soybeans and egg yolk. Food sources of lecithin include grains, legumes, fish, wheat germ and brewers yeast. I use lecithin granules derived from soybean. People who are battling serious diseases such as chronic fatigue syndrome and other immune disorders may benefit more from egg yolk lecithin according to recent studies. With this in mind, use soy lecithin for brain and cholesterol concerns and egg yolk lecithin for immune disorder conditions. For your convenience, I have listed my source for soy lecithin at the back of the book.

IMMUNE-BOOSTING HERBS

Herbs have been used for centuries to treat various conditions. Following the Immune-Boosting Herbal Remedy Chart I have listed other beneficial herbs.

IMMUNE-BOOSTING HERBAL REMEDY CHART

The following herbs have a long history of success in improving the listed sub-health conditions:

ABSCESSES
- Astragalus
- Tea tree oil

ATHLETE'S FOOT
- Goldenseal

ALZHEIMER'S DISEASE
- Gingko biloba
- Garlic

BACTERIAL INFECTIONS
- Echinacea
- Goldenseal

ANXIETY
- Chamomile
- Gotu kola
- Valerian
- Asthma
- Astragalus
- Eucalyptus

BLOOD CLOTS
- Ginseng
- Ginkgo biloba
- Garlic
- Burns
- Aloe
- Gotu kola

CANCER
- Garlic
- Siberian ginseng
- Turmeric
- Dandelion root

CONSTIPATION
- Cascara sagrada
- Ginseng
- Senna

CANKER SORES
- Goldenseal

CUTS
- Aloe

HIGH CHOLESTEROL
- Garlic
- Cayenne

DEPRESSION
- St. John's Wort

COLDS
- Echinacea
- Astragalus
- Peppermint

DIABETES
- Garlic
- Ginseng
- Goldenseal

DIGESTION
- Cayenne
- Chamomile

EARS (RINGING)
- Gingko biloba
- Peppermint

IMMUNE-BOOSTING HERBAL REMEDY CHART

HEART DISEASE
- Garlic
- Cayenne
- Hawthorn berry

LIVER PROBLEMS
- Milk thistle
- Ginseng
- Turmeric

HIGH BLOOD PRESSURE
- Feverfew
- Garlic
- Valerian

MEMORY
- Gingko biloba
- Gotu kola

IMPOTENCE
- Ginkgo biloba

MIGRAINES
- Feverfew

MOTION SICKNESS
- Ginger

NAUSEA
- Ginger

INSOMNIA
- Valerian
- Gotu kola
- Astragalus

NERVOUSNESS
- Chamomile
- Valerian
- Passionflower
- Kava kava

PAIN
- Cayenne
- Peppermint
- White willow bark

VEIN PROBLEMS
- Gotu kola
- Chamomile

PROSTATE PROBLEMS
- Saw palmetto
- Echinacea
- Goldenseal

VIRAL DISEASE
- Garlic
- Astragalus

SORE THROAT
- Goldenseal
- Licorice
- Ginger

UPSET STOMACH
- Peppermint
- Chamomile

SUNBURN
- Aloe

Aloe—God's natural bandage

For many years, I have kept an aloe plant on my kitchen window sill. Since most of my family's little cuts and scratches occur in or around the kitchen, this wonderful plant has come to the rescue more than once. I simply snip off a piece of the leaves and squeeze the thick healing gel right onto the wound. When it dries, it forms a clear natural bandage that prevents infection and promotes healing.

Aloe also can be used as a laxative and a remedy for skin rashes and eruptions. Keep in mind that aloe used as a laxative is very powerful. I prefer that you find an herbal formula that has aloe as one of its components instead of aloe alone. Also, occasionally some people have reported allergic reactions to aloe, so try it externally first. The worst that could happen is that you may develop a rash. This should disappear when you stop applying it. Aloe has been used for centuries by the Egyptians, Indians and American pioneers. Today it still proves to be one of the best remedies for cuts, burns, sunburn and skin problems.

- Softens skin
- Prevents spread of infection
- Helps heal burns and sunburn

Astragalus

This is a wonderful Chinese herb that I used in my journey to wellness. The M. D. Anderson Cancer Clinic in Houston, Texas, found that this herb may boost T-cell count in people with cancer or a lowered immune system. Yes, astragalus is making its way into health food stores all across America. When I used it years ago, it was almost unheard of in this country. The experience I had when using astragalus was remarkable. Astragalus is said to strengthen the vital energy of a weakened person. This is exactly what I experienced. I had Epstein-Barr virus, or chronic fatigue syndrome. Astragalus was just what my body needed. It also enhanced the action of all the other herbs I was consuming. Astragalus is helpful in many different health conditions, including asthma, nervousness, colds and arthritis, and especially in boosting immune function.

You may experience a little abdominal bloating when using astragalus. This is not harmful. Just cut your dosage back until the bloating disappears. This herb is very important in strengthening your entire system.

- Boosts immune system
- Protects heart from viral damage
- Heals abscesses

Cayenne

Cayenne is a really hot herb in more ways than one. This bright red herb is used extensively in many healing formulas. Cayenne actually soothes the chronic pain of arthritis, diabetic foot pain and even shingles. Most importantly, cayenne aids digestion and helps prevent heart disease. Scientists believe that cayenne, sometimes called capsaicin, assists digestion by stimulating the flow of saliva and stomach secretions. This in turn helps the digestive process. I recommend taking cayenne in capsule form, which you may buy in just about any health food store in America. I also keep a pepper shaker of cayenne on my dinner table. You don't need much to derive therapeutic benefits.

If heart disease runs in your family, or if it is a concern, cayenne cuts cholesterol levels and reduces the risk of blood clots that trigger heart attacks. According to Daniel Mowrey, Ph.D., author of *The Scientific Validation of Herbal Medicine,* cayenne is generally safe for everyone. If you have a history of ulcers, you may have a problem with cayenne. Also, be very careful not to get any cayenne in your eyes or mucous membranes, or you will definitely feel the burn. There are arthritis creams on the market that contain capsaicin. These creams feel as though they are heating up the painful area when applied. Actually, this is called counter-irritant therapy. It causes a minor discomfort to distract the user from any deeper pain. Superficially, it seems to relieve pain by this heat-producing sensation.

In addition, cayenne acts as a catalyst to enhance the effectiveness of other herbs and helps rid the body of sinus problems, sore throats and upper respiratory infections. This herb is beneficial for many health conditions.

- Reduces cholesterol
- Eases pain
- Aids digestion

Chamomile

Grandma was right about wonderful chamomile. Considered one of the world's safest herbs, chamomile helps just about anything. It relieves indigestion, calms the nerves and reduces swelling from sore muscles or bruises when applied topically. Chamomile is a traditional remedy for stress and anxiety, indigestion and insomnia. If you are allergic to ragweed, daisies or chrysanthemums, then you should avoid chamomile since it is in the same family. Chamomile has been used as a hot, soothing tea for many generations. There are, however, other ways to enjoy this time-tested herb. Chamomile extract can be purchased and added to a hot bowl of water to create a steam inhaler to unclog nasal passages. Ten to twenty drops of tincture of chamomile in water three times daily can help relieve indigestion, nervousness and menstrual cramping.

· Calms nerves
· Calms the stomach
· Relieves swelling

Echinacea

Another very effective immune system booster is my favorite herb echinacea. For years, many households in this country kept echinacea on hand as an infection fighter. That is, until the antibiotic era. Then good old echinacea became an afterthought. Thankfully, echinacea has made a grand comeback. In Germany, echinacea's infection-fighting properties are well known due to extensive research that has been done over the past few decades. Echinacea can treat colds, flu and prevent infection while bolstering the immune system. I once had a patient undergoing chemotherapy for throat cancer. After his fourth treatment, his white blood cell count dropped drastically. I recommended 20 drops echinacea liquid herbal tincture three times per day. In no time at all his count rose to normal limits. I use echinacea at the first sign of a cold or flu. Most of the time, echinacea helps my body knock out the microbes that are attacking my system. If I do wind up getting a cold or flu after taking echinacea, it is usually very short in duration. My clients agree that it really does make a difference.

If you are traveling by air, I recommend that you fortify your system with echinacea before, during and after your flight. This will boost your immune system so you won't have to battle illness on your trip, whether it be for business or a precious family vacation.

- Boosts immune system
- Helps prevent and reduce cold and flu symptoms
- Infection fighter

Goldenseal

This herb gets my seal of approval. An herb that acts as an antibiotic, cleanses the body and has anti-inflammatory and antibacterial properties, goldenseal is one of the world's most popular healing plants. What researchers know about goldenseal is that its roots contain two active components known as hydrastine and berberine. Berberine kills many bacteria, especially the ones that cause diarrhea and other infections, while boosting immune function. In addition, berberine acts as a mild pain killer, relieving many a sore throat. There is evidence that berberine can rev up the immune system by boosting white blood cells. I have used goldenseal also at the first sign of cold symptoms, and it usually stops it from developing at all.

Goldenseal is used around the world. Take it only under the supervision of a knowledgeable source such as a physician or a natural health consultant who knows about herbs. If you are pregnant or have high blood pressure, cardiovascular disease, diabetes or glaucoma, make sure to check with your physician before using goldenseal.

· Antibiotic
· Anti-inflammatory
· Boosts immune system

Saw palmetto

This herb is a godsend for men over fifty. More than half of all men in this age group will experience symptoms that indicate an enlarged prostate gland. What are the telltale symptoms that this gland is becoming a problem? First, you may have a frequent, urgent need to urinate, or you may have an interrupted urine flow or possibly trouble emptying your bladder. Drugs and surgery are routinely used to treat benign prostate hypertrophy (BPH) or enlarged prostate. Many men have decided to give saw palmetto a try before resorting to drugs or surgery. I recommend that you first go to your family doctor or urologist and make sure that you are dealing with BPH and nothing more serious, as the same symptoms can be indicative of prostate cancer. Your doctor may order a PSA test to see if your condition needs to be evaluated further. If you get the green light from your doctor, tell him you want to try saw palmetto. Most physicians are aware of its benefits. I personally know a few who take it for their own prostate health.

How does saw palmetto work? Studies in Europe show that it appears to counteract the effects of androgens, which are male hormones that stimulate prostate growth or enlargement. The recommended dosage is 320 milligrams of an oil-based extract daily. Make sure to work with your doctor so he can monitor your progress. Men report improved urinary flow, less hesitancy and a stronger flow. These results are usually noticeable after about three months of use, as with most natural supplements.

- Reduces the symptoms of prostate enlargement

St. John's Wort—nature's antidepressant

Although many experts are still studying just how it works, St. John's Wort has been shown in several studies to be just as effective at relieving symptoms of mild to moderate depression as prescription antidepressants. In addition, St. John's Wort contains antibacterial, antiviral and anti-inflammatory chemicals. One German study showed that St. John's Wort can greatly reduce the healing time of burns and also reduces scarring. This study was done involving a St. John's Wort ointment that is not currently available in the United States. But it could be available soon since this herb is one of the most popular in our country.

There are precautions that should be taken when using St. John's Wort. You should not take it with prescription antidepressants because the end result could be too much for your system. The next precaution is to be aware that St. John's Wort can make certain individuals with fair complexions more sensitive to the sun, which could result in a bad sunburn. While using St. John's Wort, you should probably avoid sun bathing or being outdoors unless you use a sunscreen with a SPF of fifteen or higher.

· Natural antidepressant
· Wound healer

Valerian—a sleep aid from heaven

Valerian has long been used to help people fall to sleep and to calm anxious minds. Valerian users claim that they wake feeling refreshed, well rested and not groggy as with prescription sleep aids. When I first used valerian, I was sure that there was some kind of mistake or that someone was playing a cruel joke on me, because it smells absolutely awful and tastes worse than that. So when you take valerian, get it in capsule form and you will have no problem. (My first experience with this herb was in a cup of hot tea. Not a pleasant experience, but it did work. I remember saying that it had better work because with a taste like that, it had better do something!) Because of its relaxing effect on the body, the following conditions are also helped by the use of valerian: irritable bowel, mucus from colds, cramps, pain, stress and ulcers.

Valerian has been shown to help women who experience menstrual cramping because it has muscle-relaxing properties. Take valerian as directed on the bottle. I prefer a valerian blend for the nervous system that not only contains valerian but also passionflower, skullcap and B vitamins. I like the synergism of herbal blend formulas. They seem to give you a more well-rounded effect. As with any herbal remedy, do not use valerian in large amounts or for a long period of time. Always remember that more is not always better. Herbs are powerful substances not to be abused. When used correctly, they are a blessing, just like all the gifts that God has given us.

· Calms the anxious
· Promotes sleep

Juicing

By now, I am sure you have heard about juicing and how beneficial it is for your body. Thanks to the "JuiceMan," millions of Americans have heard about juicing and the incredible amount of nourishment it gives our body.

Why is juicing so health promoting? Because juices extracted from fresh raw fruits and vegetables furnish all the cells in the body with the elements they need in the manner in which they can be easily assimilated.

Fruit juices are the cleansers of our bodies, and vegetable juices are the builders and regenerators of our systems. Vegetable juices contain all the minerals, salts, amino acids, enzymes and vitamins that the human body requires. This is why both fruit and vegetable juices are so important in a body-balancing immune system makeover.

Another benefit of adding juices to your immune-boosting plan is that juices are digested and assimilated within ten to fifteen minutes after consumption, and they are used almost completely by the body to nourish and regenerate the cells, tissues, glands and organs. The end result is very positive because of the minimal effort needed by the digestive system.

One of the most important things to remember

about juicing is to always drink your juices fresh daily, that is, when they are at their peak as far as nutritional value. Also, fresh juices spoil quickly, so it is better to make fresh juice daily. In addition, if you are ill or have a history of digestive difficulty, be sure to dilute your juice with water in a 50-50 mix. This way you will prevent any bloating, gas or discomfort you may experience from taking all of this liquid nutrition into your body.

As a general rule of thumb, one pint daily is the least amount needed that will show any result. When I was regaining my health, I drank two to three pints daily.

I have included some of the same formulas that I have personally used and ones that I have recommended to my clients for various sub-health conditions. Drink fruit juices at different times of the day than vegetable juices so as to prevent stomach upset.

JUICING

Wash the fruits and vegetables in ten drops of grapefruit seed extract. Be sure to scrub the fruits and vegetables with a brush to help remove any pesticide residue.

ARTHRITIS
- Grapefruit juice
- Carrot and spinach juice
- Celery juice
- Carrot and celery juice

ANEMIA
- Carrot, celery, parsley and spinach juice
- Carrot, beet and celery juice
- Carrot and spinach juice

BLADDER TROUBLE
- Carrot and spinach juice
- Carrot, beet and cucumber juice
- Carrot, celery and parsley juice

BRONCHITIS
- Carrot and spinach juice
- Carrot and dandelion juice
- Carrot, beet and cucumber juice

COLDS
- Carrot, beet and cucumber juice
- Carrot, celery and radish juice
- Carrot and spinach juice

CONSTIPATION
- Carrot and spinach juice
- Spinach juice
- Carrot juice

FATIGUE
- Carrot juice
- Carrot and spinach juice
- Carrot, beet and cucumber juice

FEVER
- Grapefruit juice
- Lemon juice
- Orange juice

GALLBLADDER AND GALLSTONES
- Carrot, beet and cucumber juice
- Carrot and spinach juice
- Carrot, celery and parsley juice

HEADACHES
- Carrot and spinach juice
- Carrot, celery, parsley and spinach juice
- Carrot, lettuce and spinach juice

INSOMNIA
- Carrot and spinach juice
- Carrot and celery juice
- Carrot, beet and cucumber juice

LIVER PROBLEMS
- Carrot, beet and cucumber juice
- Carrot and spinach juice
- Carrot juice

MENOPAUSAL SYMPTOMS
- Carrot and spinach juice
- Carrot, beet, lettuce and turnip juice

NERVOUS TENSION
- Carrot and spinach juice
- Carrot and celery juice
- Carrot, beet and cucumber juice

SCIATICA
- Carrot and spinach juice
- Carrot, spinach, turnip and watercress juice

SINUS TROUBLE
- Carrot and spinach juice
- Carrot juice
- Carrot, beet and cucumber juice

ULCERS
- Carrot and spinach juice
- Cabbage juice
- Carrot, beet and cucumber juice

Here is my favorite:

Immune-Boosting Juice Cocktail

3 carrots	1 orange
1 apple	½ beet

Juice this mixture in your juicer. Make a fresh batch every day and enjoy for an added boost.

LOVE-YOUR-LIVER FLUSH

Since your liver is one of your most important organs, special attention should be given to this hard-working filter of your body. Years ago, I was introduced to a very old procedure called the liver and gallbladder flush. This flush improves the immune system by detoxifying the liver and gallbladder. It is a powerful system rejuvenator that helps to restore the liver and gallbladder to normal function. This is done by literally flushing small gallstones out from the gallbladder and hepatic duct.

Many people with gallstones do not realize that they have them. The causes of gallstones are the inability to digest too many fatty and fried foods, indigestion from too much dairy, refined sugar, food allergies, high cholesterol sediment and hormone replacement, and lack of regular exercise. After personally performing the liver flush on myself, many stones left my body, thereby sparing me pain and discomfort that could have occurred later on. This may seem hard to believe. The truth is that this procedure has been known for many years and is routinely done by people all over the world.

Here are the instructions for the liver and gallbladder flush. (It is very important to note that this flush is not recommended for people who have had large gallstones diagnosed by their physicians. This flush is for expelling stones that range in size from a sunflower seed to a cherry pit. Anything larger could be too large to pass through the hepatic duct! So again, this is not for large stones. This is a preventative measure that is initially used to expel stones, then used periodically for maintenance.)

Monday through Saturday at noon, drink as much apple juice as you can in addition to your regular meals and any supplements you are taking. Drink only high-quality apple juice without additives. Purchase a natural juice from the health food store or juice your own organic apples. Saturday noon, eat your normal lunch. Three hours later, take 1 tablespoon of Epsom salt dissolved in ¼ cup warm water. This acts as a laxative, which will help the expulsion process. I must warn you that Epsom salt does not taste very good, so drink a little fresh grapefruit juice right after. Two hours later, repeat with 1 teaspoon of Epsom salt dissolved in ¼ cup warm water, followed by fresh grapefruit juice. For Saturday's dinner, have grapefruit juice for your meal.

At bedtime, drink ½ cup warm unrefined olive oil. I prefer extra-virgin. Blend this with ½ cup fresh lemon juice. After this, you should go directly to bed. Lie on your right side with your knees pulled up close to your chest for thirty minutes. Keep in mind that it is perfectly normal to experience nausea after drinking this olive oil mixture. It will pass as you fall asleep. The next morning, one hour before breakfast, take 1 tablespoon of Epsom salt dissolved in ¼ cup warm water. After this you may go back to your regular immune-system eating plan. When you have your next bowel movement, you should notice small gallstone-type objects in the stool. They range in color from light to dark green and in size from sunflower seeds to cherry pits. Most people find this absolutely amazing. Most skeptics become real proponents of the flush. If you see a large number of stones, the flush should be repeated in about one month. I recommend the liver flush once a year for maintenance. This flush is a very important self-treatment. When your liver is clean and functioning well, the whole body benefits. This procedure falls under the category of something that you have to see to believe. Believe me, you won't believe your eyes!

NATURAL HEALING FOR COMMON AILMENTS

Arthritis

The two most common forms of arthritis are osteo-arthritis and rheumatoid arthritis. Osteoarthritis is a wear-and-tear, age-related condition caused by friction between bones. This causes inflammation stiffness and pain. Many former athletes suffer from osteoarthritis falls due to a past of high-intensity exercise and sports activities. Rheumatoid arthritis falls under the category of an auto-immune disorder. This means that the immune system overreacts to foreign matter in the joints, causing deterioration, bone and cartilage damage, scar tissue and narrow spaces between the joints. This disease affects the entire body. The causes of rheumatoid arthritis are a genetic disposition, dietary and stress. Some women with breast implants develop rheumatoid arthritis due to the overreaction of the immune system to the foreign implant material. The most common causes of osteoarthritis are overuse of muscles, bones and joints; a deficiency in the nutrients that form collagen; and deficiencies in the nutrients that feed the muscles, ligaments and tendons.

To help alleviate arthritis symptoms from the inside out, add the following foods to your diet: apple cider vinegar, lentils, chicken and fish. Avoid the nightshade family of foods—eggplant, green peppers, tomatoes, tobacco and white potatoes. Take 500 milligrams of the enzyme bromelain twice daily between meals; 1,000 milligrams of vitamin C three times daily; 1000 milligrams of glucosamine daily; essential fatty acids; and plant enzymes to aid digestion.

Massage, detoxification, drinking plenty of water, putting warm castor oil packs over the affected area, getting some form of exercise and trying Dr. Janet's Glucosamine Cream will also help.

Bladder infections

Seventy-five percent of American women experience at least one or more urinary tract infections in a ten-year period, and 30 percent of women have one once a year. Measures must be taken quickly at the first sign of infection to prevent kidney involvement, which is more serious. Symptoms include frequent urination, low back pain, burning and cloudy urine. Common causes include stress, candida yeast infection from antibiotic overuse, food allergies and lack of adequate fluid intake to keep the body flushed.

At the first sign of infection, take all of the following until you get relief: cranberry capsules as directed, grapefruit seed extract capsules, Kyo-Dophilus probiotic formula, ACES, Kyo-Green or liquid chlorophyll.

Follow the immune eating plan, and continue to eat yeast free. Take Kyolic Garlic Extract, and drink plenty of water daily.

Chronic fatigue syndrome and Epstein-Barr Virus
Chronic fatigue syndrome and Epstein-Barr virus are the result of lowered immune function and are accompanied by yeast infections, allergies and virus activity. Many researchers believe that chronic fatigue syndrome is the result of a chronic infection with the Epstein-Barr virus, which is a latent virus that becomes active when normal immune response is compromised. I personally have battled and overcome this condition. I had to concentrate on detoxification, liver function, immune support and stress management. The immune response has to be rebuilt and supported by vitamins, minerals, herbs and most importantly, prayer.

Follow the Immune System Eating Plan with the following supplements:

- Wheat germ oil for oxygen
- B-complex vitamin
- Milk thistle
- Vitamin C crystals—¼ teaspoon every half hour to bowel tolerance to flush tissues for seven days
- Raw adrenal gland supplement
- Astragalus
- Reishi mushroom
- Liquid garlic extract—in vegetable juice daily
- Magnesium—400 milligrams at bedtime
- ACES
- Coenzyme Q_{10}—90 milligrams daily
- Eliminate sugar, caffeine, alcohol, dairy and wheat
- Take detoxifying baths
- Try valerian root for restful sleep
- Practice the MANTLE technique daily
- Stay in prayer

Hiatal hernia

This bothersome condition is caused by an opening in the diaphragm that causes a protrusion of the upper part of the stomach into the esophagus. The uncomfortable symptoms include acid reflux, burning and inflammation. The following will help to improve the quality of your life: First, eat several small meals daily; never lie down right after a meal. Avoid the following foods that aggravate the condition: coffee, sodas, tea, chocolate, lemons, tomato juice, grapefruit, oranges and spicy foods. Do not drink with your meals; wait to drink until after eating. This will help you digest your food better. Do not put ice in your beverages; this also affects digestion.

The following supplements will be a blessing: plant enzymes with each meal; Kyo-Green or liquid chlorophyll; Kyo-Dophilus or an acidophilus supplement; and chamomile tea at bedtime.

High cholesterol

Causes of high cholesterol include the following:

- Too much sugar
- Overconsumption of foods that are high in saturated fat and cholesterol, like butter, eggs, cheese, heavy cream and fatty meats
- High-stress levels—which cause an overproduction of adrenaline, which is manufactured in the adrenal glands. Most hormones, including adrenaline, are manufactured from cholesterol. Therefore, when more adrenaline is needed, more cholesterol is needed.
- Genetic predisposition
- Diuretics can raise cholesterol by causing essential minerals to be excreted. Mineral loss causes

stress on the nervous system, leading to an increased need for adrenaline.

- Estrogen and progesterone—levels of cholesterol will rise in women who have difficulty converting cholesterol to estrogen and progesterone.

Avoiding the following foods can provide a natural remedy to help lower your cholesterol:

- Sugars and saturated fats
- Cake
- Ice cream
- Pretzels
- Hot dogs
- Dairy products
- Fried or scrambled eggs
- Cookies
- Soda
- Candy
- Pizza
- Junk food
- Hamburgers
- Cream cheese

You can also take the following supplements to help lower your cholesterol:

- Lecithin—2 tablespoons of granules daily
- Garlic—500 milligrams four times daily
- Coenzyme Q_{10}—30 milligrams three times a day
- Fish oil—2,000 milligrams (salmon)
- Vitamin C—1,000 milligrams three times daily
- Choline, inositol—daily as directed
- Carnitine—500 milligrams twice daily
- Shiitake or reishi mushrooms—as directed
- Red yeast rice—blood lipid formula
- Chromium picolinate—as directed
- Apple pectin

Continue to follow the Immune System Eating Plan. Oat bran and brown rice are especially good for lowering cholesterol.

1. *Follow the immune eating plan with added recipes.*
2. *Recommended supplements:*
   - Carlson Multivitamin and Mineral Gelcaps
   - Green drink daily: Kyo-Green by Wakunaga
   - Bragg's Liquid Aminos on foods
   - Extra-virgin olive oil
   - Antioxidants daily: Carlson ACES
   - Stevia extract instead of artificial sweeteners
   - Calcium/magnesium supplement daily: CalMax powder
   - B-complex vitamin with extra pantothenic acid
   - 200 mcg. of chromium daily (over 150 pounds, take 400 mcg.)
3. *Immune boosters: choose one or more*
   - Astragalus
   - Echinachea
   - Maitake/Shiitake/Reishi mushrooms
4. *Natural antibiotics: choose one*
   - Biotic silver
   - Olive leaf extract
   - Grapefruit seed extract
   - Goldenseal
5. *Heart health: choose one or more*
   - Coenzyme Q_{10}
   - Hawthorn berry
   - L-Carnitine
   - CalMax powder
   - Garlic or Kyolic EPA
6. *High cholesterol: choose one or more*
   - Red yeast rice
   - Lecithin granules
   - Guggul
   - Garlic
   - Chromium
   - Fiber
   - Choline, Inositol
   - Vitamin C
7. *Stress: choose one or more*
   - CalMax powder
   - B complex
   - ACES
   - Reishi mushrooms
   - Chamomile
   - Astragalus
   - Kava kava
   - Valerian
   - Wild American ginseng
   - Massage
   - Baths
   - Prayer
8. *Blood sugar balance: choose one or more*
   - Chromium picolinate
   - Fiber
   - Stevia extract
   - Kyo-Green
   - B complex
9. *Drink enough water, get sufficient sleep and pray daily.*
10. *Detoxify twice a year—spring and fall.*

Three Ways to Enhance Your Makeover Result

I am very excited to share with you three wonderful products to enhance your new higher level of health: progesterone cream, glucosamine cream and skin cream.

Progesterone cream

After struggling for twenty years with severe hormonal imbalance and discovering the reason was an imbalance in my estrogen-progesterone ratio, I am pleased to share with you my formula birthed out of my own quest for hormonal balance and well-being. I call it Dr. Janet's Balanced by Nature Progesterone Cream. It contains pure pharmaceutical-grade natural progesterone derived from the Mexican wild yam. In addition, it meets the specifications that John Lee, M.D., recommends for an effective cream. I have included the product information and description for you.

If you can't lose weight or are experiencing cramps, migraines, bloating, breast tenderness, hot flashes, lack of energy, depression, mood swings, fibroid tumors, endometriosis, infertility, family history female-related cancer, foggy thinking, perimenopause, or losing height, you may be experiencing hormonal imbalance. Dr. Janet's Balanced by Nature Progesterone Cream can help cramps, bloating, depression, mood swings, water retention, hot flashes and decreased libido, can prevent osteoporosis, and protect against breast fibroids.

Everyone is different. As such, the use of natural progesterone body cream should be adjusted to meet your own needs. The following suggestions are to be used as a guide only. Although there have been no reports of any significant side effects or health problems associated with natural progesterone, consider consulting your physician. Some women notice results right away, while others may see changes in one to three months.

Use the progesterone cream between ovulation until the onset of menses (the time of ovulation can be determined by a dramatic change—rise or fall—in basal body temperature and by changes, thinning or thickening, in vaginal secretions). Some women also experience lower abdominal pains during ovulation. If you have symptoms prior to ovulation (for example, migraines), you may want to begin using the cream earlier, until your period. You don't need natural progesterone during menstruation. However, if you experience cramps or other symptoms during menstruation, you may use the cream until the symptoms are alleviated.

For PMS and menopausal symptoms: After ovulation (days 14–18 after onset of last period), use small amount of cream, no more than ¼ teaspoon once a day. Days 18–23, use ¼ teaspoon twice daily, gradually increasing to ½ teaspoon twice daily. Day 23 until period, use ½ teaspoon twice daily.

For osteoporosis: Bone density testing is recommended before using natural progesterone. This is to establish a baseline from which to measure changes in your bone density every six to twelve months. Consult your health care provider. Use ¼ teaspoon to ½ teaspoon (for severe cases) daily.

For postmenopausal: Use cream for three weeks, ¼ to ½ teaspoon twice per day. Go one week without cream.

Please note that while low-dose natural progesterone creams are generally effective for mild PMS symptoms, it has been found that higher doses (980–1000 mg. per 2–oz. jar) of natural progesterone cream have been more effective in balancing a woman's system during premenopause, menopause and postmenopause. This is especially true for the prevention and treatment of osteoporosis.

Glucosamine cream

Arthritis can be a real pain! I have developed a pain relief cream for arthritis that contains all of the cutting-edge ingredients currently getting a lot of press for their effectiveness. I pass a jar of this unique formulation around to my audience during seminars. I instruct anyone who is in pain from arthritis, muscle pain, injury and even fibromyalgia to apply this cream. At the fifteen-minute break, I ask how many people are still hurting. Remarkably, almost everyone has gotten relief.

Glucosamine cream is a specially blended combination of all natural ingredients, listed as follows:

Emu oil. This oil, as scientific studies have shown, was used thousands of years ago by Australian aborigines, who found this versatile bird to be a valuable resource for natural, effective solutions to many of their most basic problems, such as food, clothing, shelter and relief from pain. Muscle pain, sunburn pain and inflammation in the joints can be relieved as a result of two substances that occur naturally in the oil itself: lenolenic acid (the pain killer) and oleic acid (an anti-inflammatory).

The natural properties of the emu oil are so simple

and non-intrusive that our skin has no need for resistance to it. Therefore, the oil is permitted to simply pass through the skin layer without interruption, providing the immediate benefit—pain relief—for you!

Pregnenolone. Pregnenolone is a natural hormone produced by the body when cholesterol is broken down in the mitochondria of the cell. This remarkable process occurs naturally in the brain and adrenal glands. Scientific and medical studies have shown that as we age, our levels of pregnenolone decline, although the continued balance of natural hormones, such as pregnenolone, is essential to our optimum good health. While pregnenolone is not found naturally in plants, it can be manufactured naturally from plants. The wild yam, native to Mexico and China, is a common and reliable source for natural pregnenolone production.

Used successfully for more than fifty years for the effective relief of the pain and inflammation of arthritis, pregnenolone also helps reduce the swelling and stiffness associated with arthritis pain. Studies have shown that the use of natural pregnenolone supplement also contributes to significant improvement in memory, task performance and a general sense of well-being.

Glucosamine sulfate. Glucosamine sulfate is a substance found naturally in your body. It is a combination of sugar and amine. As a natural constituent of cartilage that stimulates the production of connective tissue in your body, glucosamine production slows in the body as we age, leaving the cartilage unable to retain water and thereby reducing the "shock-absorber" effect we enjoyed with healthier cartilage when proper levels were naturally produced by the body. Glucosamine sulfate works to lubricate your joints, rebuilds damaged cartilage and stimulates the production of new cartilage.

Boswellin. Boswellin is a natural extract from the herb boswellia, used as an ancient natural remedy for arthritis sufferers. It is now widely acknowledged for its cutting-edge benefits and effectiveness for the relief of arthritis pain and inflammation.

Bromelain. Bromelain, an enzyme derived from pineapple juice, blocks inflammation by stimulating the production of plasmin, a body compound that aids the reduction of localized swelling.

No capsaicin is used. No extract of hot pepper or cayenne means no burning sensation to the skin! Dr. Janet's Balanced by Nature Glucosamine Cream provides relief from arthritis pain without discomfort.

Balanced by Nature products are made with the highest grade of quality ingredients; only the most expensive oils, virtually odorless and colorless, are used. This high-quality formulation of emu oil, pregnenolone and glucosamine sulfate, along with proper amounts of specially selected herbs, vitamins and enzymes, is the product of years of study and research. It was developed for natural, effective solutions for my clients' continued good health. This has been the goal as well as the result. Blended with a specially formulated cream base, Balanced by Nature Glucosamine Cream is the solution I recommend to my clients for relief of arthritis symptoms because it works naturally to ease their pain and inflammation from arthritis. Apply the glucosamine cream by placing a small amount, approximately ¼ to ½ teaspoon of cream, on your fingertips and rub gently into the area of your pain, directly onto the skin. If your arthritis pain is located in your joints or covered by a large amount of tissue (hips, thighs or shoulders), simply increase the amount of cream and apply more generously directly to the joint area. The cream should penetrate. Relief begins within a minute.

Skin cream

Many times after a person goes through the immune makeover program, they feel so great that they begin to focus on their outward appearance again.

Appearance is not everything, nor is vanity a desirable attribute. It is a barometer that I use as a confirmation that a person is well and ready to face the world again. So to me, it's a very good sign.

I have helped to develop a skin cream formulated with collagen, elastin, antioxidants and stevia in a base that is so absorbable and healing to the skin that people from all over the country do not want to be without it. Dr. Janet's Balanced by Nature Skin Cream is a special formulation of safe, effective and natural ingredients.

Elastin CLR. Elastin CLR is an innovative active ingredient. It has been clinically studied and consumer-tested in its effectiveness on diseased and damaged skin tissue. Published clinical studies indicated that Elastin CLR, serving as a natural building material, can provide a reliable foundation for the development of new, healthy skin tissue. Think of it as an efficient health program for your skin. Elastin CLR builds and strengthens the structure of the very fibers of your skin tissue while regenerating growth of new skin tissue in replacement of existing damaged and diseased tissue. The more obvious results are readily apparent in the epidermal layer of the skin. Wrinkles, scar tissue and scaliness can be minimized.

By promoting increased moisture binding in existing skin fibers and generating the formation of healthier, new elastin fibers in the skin, Elastin CLR has attendant benefits for skin that is currently unhealthy or healthy. You can see the difference! Elastin CLR has an extended shelf life and is nontoxic.

Papaya. Papaya contains a proteolytic enzyme known as papain, which serves as a natural enzymatic exfoliant.

Stevia extract. Stevia extract, also known as "sweet herb," has been used for centuries as the antibacterial agent in skin care treatments. So safe, stevia is also edible, an excellent natural sugar substitute.

Collagen CLR, natural glycerine, calcium, natural oils and vitamins A, E, B$_3$, B$_6$ and D. Collagen CLR, natural glycerine, calcium, natural oils and vitamins A, E, B$_3$, B$_6$ and D are among the other all-natural ingredients that have been carefully selected and blended to create this very unique skin cream.

Unlike other elastin products, Dr. Janet's Balanced by Nature Skin Cream, using the proper combination of highest quality and grade ingredients available, delivers a product designed for long-lasting as well as immediately healthier skin results.

Dr. Janet's Balanced by Nature Skin Cream is formulated with 10 percent elastin and 4 percent collagen to restore elasticity and tone. Surface lines and wrinkles will be replaced with a smoother and firmer appearance as nourishing moisturizers restore the moisture balance. The result…your skin will be more supple, more youthful and naturally radiant!

There are no known side effects associated with these products. Years of studies—medical and scientific as well as extensive consumer use—have shown safe, effective skin care results are available to you the Balanced by Nature way.

Dr. Janet's Balanced by Nature Skin Cream contains no acids and is so easy to apply. Simply place a small amount on your fingertips and smooth gently into your skin. The cream will penetrate your skin immediately, is easily absorbed and leaves no unpleasant residue. It is versatile enough for day time use, even under makeup, or diligent as a nighttime vitamin boost while you sleep.

So gentle, it is non-irritating to your eyes and the more delicate tissue around your eyes. It will not clog pores and can be used by those with sensitive skin. It is recommended for all skin types and has been shown to:

- Heal and restore moisture
- Rebuild natural tissue elastin
- Restructure fine-line skin fiber
- Smooth existing fine lines
- Minimize wrinkles
- Provide psoriasis relief
- Repair sun-wrinkled skin
- Lighten brown age spots
- Rejuvenate facial skin
- Promote the decline of wrinkles
- Promote moisture binding in the skin
- Promote formation of new elastin fibers in the skin
- Improve the healing process of postoperative wounds

- Reduce inflammation
- Protect against skin irritations
- Have positive effects on damaged or diseased skin
- Soften and smooth keloids
- Improve the texture of your skin
- Cause realignment of facial tissue fiber
- Rebuild elastin for healthy skin tissue

Experience the difference healthy skin, "Balanced by Nature," can make in your life, the way you look and the way you feel about your appearance...naturally!

EPILOGUE

━━━━━━━━━━━━━━━━ ■ ━━━━━━━━━━━━━━━━

HOSPITALS, HOLLYWOOD
AND HEALING

At the beginning of the *90-Day Immune System Makeover,* you read my story. Well, I failed to include the last part, which I have saved until now. Remember how my dream was to someday have a career in television? God truly is faithful to give us the desires of our heart—only according to His timing, not ours. Years ago when I was struggling with my health, I gave up on the aspirations of my younger days. I really almost gave up entirely.

One evening, after a series of medical tests, I had a fever and could not sleep. I went downstairs to just be alone and pray and wonder why God was allowing me to go through this wilderness experience. I picked up a magazine and noticed an ad that asked, "Could you be the next Breck Woman of the Nineties?"

I laughed to myself. It was 1989, and I did not even know if I was going to be alive in the nineties at the rate my health was going downhill. The ad continued by asking, "What would you like to see happen for women in the nineties? Tell us your thoughts in the form of an essay. Attach a picture of yourself, and you could be selected."

I really can't explain to you why I reached for a pen and piece of paper and began feverishly writing. As I wrote to the people at Breck, I poured out my heart about how women in the eighties had sacrificed so much of themselves to achieve almost impossible goals and how they felt that they had to be supermom, superwife, super everything. They climbed the top of the corporate ladder, only to find that they could be instantly and easily replaced. In the meantime, their precious opportunity to bear a child and to build a home and family was placed on the back burner to be "accomplished" at a later time. As a result, women in the eighties were tired, disillusioned, lonely and burnt out. I know, because I too was burnt out. I continued the essay by saying women in the nineties will have come full circle. They have proved that they could "make it" in the work force. Now the pressure was off. The most important job a woman could ever hold is to be a loving wife, mother and friend. She should enrich the lives of everyone with whom she comes in contact. God did not create woman to be stressed, sick, angry and lonely.

I then asked my husband to mail the letter and told him, "I have something to tell women; I just have to be heard." I attached a photo of myself as a little girl holding a bottle of Breck shampoo (it was my favorite) and a current picture of myself. Exactly one year later, after I regained my health, the telephone rang. It was Breck asking me to fly to Los Angeles to be on ABC's

Home Show for one week. I was chosen along with three other women from across the country to compete on national TV for the title of "Breck Woman of the Nineties."

There was that word *compete* again. That sounded like the same old pressure that I had sworn off, coming into the picture once again. I decided to go anyway with a new outlook because I had been transformed during my illness; the old desires passed away, and my goals were different. I flew to L.A. not feeling stressed, but victorious in my own way. Just one year before, I was ill and could hardly function. This year I was flying to Hollywood. I'm not going to bore you with all of the details. It was a wonderful experience but what I want to tell you is, yes, I became a "Breck Woman of the Nineties," but it meant nothing to me. Years ago I would have been flying high. Instead, when I was with the cast and crew of the *Home Show,* all I could talk about was how to help them feel better. I gave advice on vitamins and herbs, and I told them how I overcame chronic fatigue syndrome. The people from Breck were afraid that all I would talk about was health and not shampoo! It was at that point in time I said, "Lord, now I understand. You have given me a gift more precious than anything of this world. You have given me a healing ministry. You allowed me to walk through the fire so You could refine me. Only then could people see Your face in me and allow me to minister health to their bodies."

Once I caught God's vision for my life, I went to school and received a Ph.D. in nutrition and a degree in natural medicine, and the doors opened. God flooded me with wonderful opportunities in television, radio and seminars to reach out and help His people reclaim their health. This book is dedicated to that vision as we occupy until He comes. May God bless you.

TESTIMONIALS

VICTORY!

The following section is filled with actual case histories submitted by my clients in order to share with you their personal journey to higher immune health and well-being.

Thanks be to God, which giveth us the victory through our Lord Jesus Christ.

—1 CORINTHIANS 15:57

I first went to Dr. Janet Maccaro in July of 1997. I had been living with several difficult health problems and just could not self-prescribe any longer.

I was allergic to three different cholesterol medicines and had a cholesterol of 284. For several years I was up every night with terrible heartburn, and I had several extremely painful gout attacks. I was also very tired all the time and had very little energy. I was overweight, but I did not consider that to be my primary health problem since I was so sick of diets.

I brought my blood work results to Dr. Maccaro, told her about myself and found it very easy to relate to her. The next visit Dr. Maccaro outlined a different lifestyle for me. I did wait another week to start until I was able one day to say, "Now I am ready to take care of myself and feel better."

For me it was definitely a different way of eating, but because Dr. Maccaro told me it would make me feel better, I tried it. Now it is simply my way of life, and I have very little trouble following this lifestyle. Certainly, there are times when I have some problems, but Dr. Maccaro has been there to help me along the way either on the phone or by appointment.

Five months after I started, at my annual physical my family doctor was amazed and delighted with the new me. My cholesterol was down to 204 and my weight was down thirty pounds. To use a trite phrase, I looked and felt like a new person! I have never had another gout attack and do not get up at night with heartburn. Because I have an increased energy level, I find life to be interesting and fun.

I have been through unrelated surgery and recuperation since I first started with Dr. Maccaro, and she was there for me by phone to suggest things to help me along. I have traveled to foreign countries and was still able to follow my eating and health plan with some extra advice from Dr. Maccaro.

I lead a very active social life, and of course, friends and acquaintances have noticed the change in my attitude and appearance and question me about it. I tell all of them I could not have done any of it without the wonderful advice and help of Dr. Janet Maccaro.

—Marilyn Petrie
Ormond Beach, Florida

Five years ago, I was diagnosed with connective tissue arthritis. My whole body was so full of inflammation, I could barely move. The doctor put me on steroids (prednisone) for over a year. I also tried every prescription drug there was for my condition. Each medication had a different side effect on me. One medication sent me to the hospital's emergency room because I couldn't breathe. The doctors also put me on hormones, from which I gained twenty pounds. I was so sick I couldn't function. Two years ago, I thought my body was dying. I was so tired, breathing was an effort.

A friend of my sons gave me Dr. Janet Maccaro's phone number. He thought she might be able to help me. I called her that day and made an appointment to see her. We talked about my health problems, and she assured me that she could help me. Dr. Janet put me on a healthy eating plan and recommended vitamin supplements that could help my condition. I followed her plan to the letter because I was so anxious to get control of what was happening to my body. In about two to three months, I could feel the difference. I had more energy, and the pain was easing up.

It's been two years now. I am a happy, functioning person. I will never be pain free, but it's at a point that I can handle it. Thanks to Dr. Janet for giving me back my life. I thanked God that day I met her. She's a very special, caring person. What my doctors couldn't do for me with all their prescription drugs, Dr. Janet did with a healthy eating plan. As an added bonus, I lost forty-two pounds. I want to thank you very much for being there when I needed you.

—ELLIE KLEM
ORMOND BY THE SEA, FLORIDA

I had been searching on my own, after taking Premarin for over fifteen years, to find a natural product that would be beneficial to and address my specific needs and desire to decrease my dependence on artificial hormones. I had been fortunate to have been exposed to Dr. John Lee's film on progesterone, which led me to read his book, further enhancing my desire for a natural solution to my sluggishness and "brain fog."

I was delighted when I tuned into *Today's Family* to hear Dr. Janet speaking about natural progesterone and other natural products to put your body in balance as nature intended. Eager to learn more, I ordered her tape series. They were a great source of information that answered many of my questions.

I began following Dr. Janet's prescription for balanced health through a program of natural vitamins, supplements and natural progesterone. After approximately three months, I began to feel better overall. It was great to know, by my own experience, that I was on the right path.

I was experiencing pain in my hip, which would often wake me at night. Dr. Janet's glucosamine cream helped alleviate the pain and allowed me to go back to sleep. After a period of time, I didn't need to use it as often as the benefits built up in my body, allowing for natural healing.

I appreciate her diligence and dedication to her profession. After achieving such wonderful results for myself, I shared Dr. Janet's tapes with my sisters and friends. They have also experienced improvement in their overall health. It has truly been a blessing to me and my family that I "discovered" Dr. Janet on television. She has become a great source of information and guidance to me, my family and friends. I'm sure she would agree, as in all facets of life, that balance is the key.

(If you have the opportunity to try Dr. Janet's Skin Cream—do it! It is a wonderful moisturizer. I have seen an improvement in the texture of my face and, most notably, the area around my eyes. It is rich, smooth and creamy—a little goes a long way. This is NOT a commercial; it's the truth.)

—BRENDA AKINS
BUNNELL, FLORIDA

Words cannot express to you how much of a difference you and your wisdom have made for me! With your cleansing and weight-loss plan, I've lost at least fifteen pounds in six weeks, have more energy than ever and feel absolutely wonderful. I've shared your materials with many friends, and they love it, too! Your kindness, understanding and knowledge have changed my life.

Thank you from the bottom of my heart!

—LESA BUCKLER
LOUISVILLE, KENTUCKY

After twenty-one years of experiencing heartburn, I am now heartburn free and have been so for a year. I am, after completing your program, convinced that candida overgrowth is what killed my mom. Mom had surgery for a bowel obstruction in 1962, after which she developed a bad staph infection, was hospitalized and given massive antibiotic therapy. Within a year she was experiencing heartburn ongoingly. This lead to spontaneous vomiting, esophageal scarring and stricture to the point of being unable to eat much except liquids. She became near skeletal and ultimately suffered a heart attack brought on by malnourishment. When she got cancer of the lung, her nutritional status was so poor that they couldn't operate on her. She died nine months later. She suffered from thrush for at least six years prior to her death.

My heartburn began in 1978 and was diagnosed as stress related as a result of my divorce. I now recognize the actual cause and can trace it to a bout with septic shock in 1976, during which I was also given massive doses of antibiotics. After that I began experiencing frequent bouts of vaginitis and "honeymoon" cystitis. I was working as a recovery room nurse at that time, and I remember one of the doctors saying that "we girls got it from one another." Within a year I was the OR supervisor and having terrible heartburn.

Over the next twenty years this condition progressed to the point I could have no caffeine, no carbonated beverages, no spicy food, no alcoholic beverages—and still had heartburn daily. I lived with the large bottle of Tums in my purse, my briefcase, my kitchen and my desk. I went through a large bottle to Tums every week—and I still had heartburn! At times, for no reason, I would be struck with severe salivation and an overwhelming need to vomit. I began to see a pattern. This was progressing just like my mom! I called on my GI clients who put me on Prilosec. Heaven descended! No more heartburn—until I went off it. I tried Tagamet and other over-the-counter drugs, with varying success, but I realized I was treating symptoms not pathology. I had an *H. Pylori* test done. It was negative. I scheduled myself for an upper GI endoscopy, fearing Barrett's esophagitis. In the meantime, I noticed I was having severe premenstrual bloating. I had also noticed that the heartburn seemed to get worse whenever I ate sugar, and I had told both of my GI specialists about this possible connection. I craved sugar like a smoker craves nicotine and an alcoholic craves booze. Then, I ran into my friend and hairdresser, who looked wonderful. He told me about Dr. Janet and this whole yeast/candida theory. I called her the next day.

After going on the candida cleansing diet for one week, I was down to an occasional heartburn episode. By the end of two weeks these were rare. They were virtually gone by the end of the first month, as was the bloating and craving. The second month I did the cleansing diet. The diet was easy to follow, though for the first time in my life I had to think about the food I was putting in my body. I learned to shop at health food stores and fell in love with millet bread and crackers. Going off wheat and dairy was no problem. Rice milk and ice cream were a treat, though I had to learn to read labels carefully.

By the time I came to see Dr. Janet at the end of the second month, I had lost forty-five pounds seemingly effortlessly. I felt and looked great.

It's been a year now. I do occasionally eat sugar and recognize one bite leads me to a binge. I don't eat dairy except for cheese, which I seem to tolerate, but I have trouble with milk, so I largely don't do it. I don't eat wheat, but if I slip, I do get a bad stomachache, diarrhea and bloating, especially if the wheat is combined with sugar.

Thank you so much, Janet. You've made such a difference in my life.

—ANNE DEAN
DELAND, FLORIDA

■

Ever since I was a little girl I seemed to be sick more often than my brother and two sisters. I participated in extracurricular activities, basketball, track, band and softball, but almost every year I would get sick with tonsillitis, appendicitis, pneumonia, strep throat or something and have to be admitted to the hospital, or stay at home. The doctor would prescribe antibiotics, I would get well, and a vicious cycle would begin again.

As I grew into adulthood I remained rather sickly. Still, I married and had three children. The pregnancies were very hard on my body. Eight out of the nine months I would regurgitate severely. My body became dehydrated often, and when they would call the doctor, he would say to take me to the emergency room. In the ER they would feed me through tubes, send me home to my own bed, only to have me return again and again.

After eight years and three difficult pregnancies, my body was weak from being compromised and challenged. So I did all I could to strengthen it. I lifted weights, jogged, did aerobics and otherwise stayed active. As much as I tried to get my body to strengthen, the more it seemed to be slipping away from me.

I relocated to Orlando, Florida, and with the relocation came the task of finding a new doctor. Unfortunately, the doctor I selected made a serious mistake. I did not find out for nearly a year that instead of giving me the proper doses of hormones for my HRT (hormone replacement therapy), I was given twice the amount that my body needed. Within a few months of this treatment, I began having severe headaches. For

245

this, another doctor adjusted my spine, with no relief, and a neurologist found nothing to be causing my headaches. He suggested an MRI, for he seemed to think I had either a pinched nerve or a brain tumor. The MRI proved negative, and my headaches became worse.

My relatives suggested I see a dentist to check for TMJ dysfunction (a condition of the jaw that may cause headaches). I got a positive diagnosis, and a TMJ appliance was crafted to give my jaw the separation it needed to get the pressure off the joint. For a while it seemed as if my health was improving. The headaches subsided; I started attending college and worked.

In my second year of college, my body started breaking down again with bouts of the flu and viral pneumonia. I was admitted to the hospital to check out the lungs and the headaches again. My doctor ordered a spinal tap, which proved negative. I was sent home fighting a fever of about 102 to 103; they admitted the infection was of unknown origin. The doctor ordered intravenous broad spectrum antibiotics. They took x-rays and discovered that the infection almost killed me. Pneumonia had already settled in one lung and started in the other.

My education had to be put on hold; I did continue to work, but I started searching for other methodologies to relieve the ever-present pain and discomfort. Now, it was no longer just headaches, but pain was all over my body. I began acupuncture, which eventually didn't help.

The pain was becoming more intense; I went to several doctors to find an answer, but again no answers or relief. In July of 1995, I was so weak that I couldn't get out of bed. Walking was a problem, holding a toothbrush was a problem, and soon depression was another battle.

In desperation, I went to Jacksonville's Mayo Clinic; the rheumatologist diagnosed me with fibromyalgia. They prescribed medications to deal with this non-life-threatening but life-altering disease.

My younger sister told me of a nutritionist she came across on the Family Channel, Dr. Janet Maccaro of Ormond

Beach. Although I didn't believe holistic nutrition could help me when the medical field could not, my family and a close friend encouraged me to see Dr. Maccaro. After Dr. Maccaro did a profile on me, she was sure she could help me.

She explained about candida and how an overabundance of yeast in the body could cause the multitude of problems I had been experiencing. My health issues—high blood pressure, hyperthyroidism, spleenectomy, heart murmur, irritable bowel syndrome, allergies, Raynaud's disease, recurrent urinary/yeast and kidney infections, TMJ, dizziness, asthma, depression and still more—could be explained by Dr. Maccaro. No one had ever given so much of their time and themselves as this person discussing my health. She explained everything in layman's terms and encouraged me to have faith and to commit to this new way of life.

My program consisted of three parts: eliminate candida, internal body cleansing and an eating plan with supplementation. I found it particularly difficult to be strict with my diet, but I wanted to have my life back. After a few weeks my coworkers would stop in the hallway and tell me how much better I looked. I had a light bounce in my step, light back in my eyes and laughter came easy. The depression lifted, and I began to feel alive. Life became enjoyable again.

I still have flareups, but it is nothing compared to what my life was like before Dr. Maccaro's program. I eat healthier and rest more deeply, and I discovered life is all about choices. I choose to live. My gratitude goes out to Dr. Maccaro, who in essence gave my life back to me.

—SHIRLEY TOWNSEND
PALM COAST, FLORIDA

■

In May of 1998, my mom died of colon cancer. A few months later my sister had her colon removed as a preventative because she was experiencing diarrhea and constipation, which resulted in bloating, hemorrhoids and a plethora of other problems. It was while my sister was

247

under the influence of tranquilizers that they gave her in the hospital that she agreed to surgery and the removal of her large intestine rather than experience something she "may" have to deal with in the future. Her road to recovery has been slow and uncertain, and even now she isolates herself because of the bag she will wear for the rest of her life.

During this time, I was experiencing terrible gastrointestinal problems. I would eat one bite of a sandwich and swell up like a balloon. I too experienced diarrhea one day and constipation the next, and the pains in my stomach were scaring me to death. I knew with all certainty that I would not take the road my sister had traveled, but I had to do something. I started reading everything I could find, and as I self-diagnosed, I became more and more confused. Then one day Janet Maccaro walked into the health food store where I work; that was the day my recovery began.

Some of the things Janet told me I had heard or read about before, but I guess this is one of those "when the student is ready" things, because when I heard them that day, it was like a revelation. Eliminate wheat and sugar and supplement my diet with a really good liquid acidophilus. That's not all Janet told me that first day, but that's what I heard loud and clear. Could it be that simple? Compared to the nightmare I imagined ahead of me, I knew I could deal with food allergies.

I began immediately, and within days my symptoms disappeared, returning only when I misbehaved. One relapse was the result of eating a slice of pizza on the Fourth of July. Another time I couldn't resist the croissants at a bakery in St. Augustine. Usually within minutes after indulging I would swell up from right under my bra to my belly button, and the pain and cramping would begin, sometimes lasting for hours; it wasn't my imagination. It didn't take too many relapses for me to become convinced completely and to make a commitment to my new lifestyle. Avoiding sugar actually helped eliminate my cravings for the breads and pastas I have loved all my life, and after the first week or so, it hasn't really been difficult. Each time I resist a temptation, I think about Mom and my sister. The food I replace temptations with, like salads and proteins, taste even better to me today than the bad stuff used to taste.

As time went on, I supplemented my diet with other good things Janet has told me about, and these too have added to my recovery. One of these is Janet's progesterone cream, which has been an answer to prayer. The hot flashes are gone, and instead of that feeling of impending doom I used to have, I have a feeling of well-being. Friends tell me that I glow, and I've received the joy back in my life that I thought I'd lost somewhere in my thirties. I am a brand-new grandmother, and yet at fifty-four years old, I have more energy than ever, enough to baby-sit my bundle of joy several times a week and still keep up with almost everything else.

Good things often come with bad. Had I not been experiencing the intestinal problems, I never would have talked to Janet, because I thought the menopausal symptoms were just part of being older. Janet gave me so much that very first day, and the best thing she continues to give me is hope.

—BEST WISHES WITH THIS WONDERFUL ENDEAVOR,
SANDY WISHNOW

APPENDIX A

REFERENCES, RESOURCES AND SUGGESTED READING

Over the years many teachers, authors, lecturers and publications have been instrumental in my healing process. The following list contains information on the many references, products and contacts that I have used and highly recommend.

THE FIRST 30 DAYS

"Sugar's Effect on Insulin Levels," *American Journal of Clinical Nutrition*, 1977, p. 613.

"A Low-Fat Diet May Boost Killer Cells," *American Journal of Clinical Nutrition*, volume 50, pp. 851–867.

Balch, James, M.D. and Balch, Phyllis. *Rx for Cooking and Dietary Wellness*. PAB Books, Inc., 1992.

Black, Dean, Ph.D. *Regeneration: China's Ancient Gift to the Modern Quest for Health*, Bioresearch Foundation, 1988.

Energy Times Magazine, November/December 1999.

Fuller, Dicqie, Ph.D., D.Sc. *The Healing Power of Enzymes.* New York: Forbes Custom Publishing, 1998.

"Stress and Lower Immunity," *Lancet,* 1977, pp. 834–836.

Page, Linda Rector, N.D., Ph.D. *Healthy Healing,* ninth edition. Healthy Healing Publications.

Serafini, M. "Red Wine, Tea and Antioxidants." *Lancet,* 1994.

Stamets, Paul. *Growing Gourmet and Medicinal Mushrooms.* Ten Speed Publishing, 1994.

The Townsend Letter, June 1998.

Yang, C. S. and Wang, Z. Y. "Tea and Cancer." *Journal National Cancer Institute,* 85(13), 1038–1049.

THE NEXT 60 DAYS

Airola, Paavo, Ph.D., N.D. *Every Woman's Book,* 10th printing. Phoenix, AZ: Health Plus Publishers, 1992.

Balch, James, M.D., and Balch, Phyllis, M.D. *Prescription for Nutritional Healing.* Garden City Park, New York: Avery Publishing Group, 1997.

Barnes, Broda O., M.D. and Galton, Lawrence. *Hypothyroidism: The Unsuspected Illness.* New York: Cromwell, 1976.

"The Candida Yeast Answer Booklet." Candida Wellness Center, Gary Carlson, director. 4365 N. Bedford Drive., Provo, UT 84604. (800) 869-1613; Web site: www.candidayeast.com.

Contreras, Francisco, M.D. *Health in the 21st Century: Will Doctors Survive?* Chula Vista, CA: Interpacific Press, 1997.

Crook, W. G., M.D. *The Yeast Connection*, first edition. Jackson, TN: Professional Books, 1983.

Gagnon, Daniel O. *Healing Herbs for Your Nervous System.* Santa Fe, NM: Santa Fe Botanical Research and Educational Project, 1992.

Kaufman, Leslie. "Your Prescription Is Ready." *Health Magazine*, October 1997.

Lee, John R., M.D. *What Your Doctor May Not Tell You About Menopause.* Warner Books, 1996.

Mamadou, M., Dr. "The White Paper," *Oral Enzymes: Facts and Concepts.* Transformation Enzyme Corp., 2900 Wilcrest Blvd., Suite 220, Houston, TX 77042. (713) 266-2117.

"Medicine in the New Millennium." *The Daytona Beach News Journal*, January 22, 2000.

Peat, Raymond, M.A., Ph.D. "Hormonal Changes in Stress and Aging" (paper).

Sahley, Billie Jay, Ph.D. *Anxiety Epidemic.* San Antonio, TX: Pain and Stress Publications, 1997.

"Say Amen for Your Health's Sake." *Health Magazine*, October 1997.

Seyle, Hans. *Stress Without Distress.* New York: New American Library, 1995.

"Therapeutic Enzymes...the Energy of Life," product resource and information booklet. Enzymedica. www.enzymedica. com.

Truss, C. O., M.D. *The Missing Diagnosis.* P. O. Box 26508, Birmingham, AL 35226.

90 Days

"Antibiotic-Resistant Bacteria Spreads." *Energy Times Magazine*, November/December 1989.

Bethel Ministries, Inc., P. O. Box 150, Daytona Beach, FL 32115. (904) 672-0250. E-mail: Bethelmin@aol.com. John Jeyseelan, president and CEO. Bethel Ministries, founded in 1989, is a global evangelical organization committed to prayer, preaching and teaching of the gospel of Jesus Christ. Internationally, this mission is accomplished through worldwide crusades with the help of foreign missionaries and the training of nationals to reach the lost within their own countries. Bethel Ministries also sponsors the building of churches, feeding and education of orphan children and the financial support of foreign missionaries. Domestically, Bethel Ministries is committed to the ministry of reconciliation, unity and godly love in the body of Christ. It actively sponsors city-wide prayer gatherings in the Central Florida area.

Blumert, Michael and Liu, Jialiu, Dr. *Jiaogulan: China's Immortality Herb.* Torchlight Publishing, Inc., 1999.

Duke, James A., Ph.D. *The Green Pharmacy: New Discoveries in Herbal Remedies for Common Diseases and Conditions From the World's Foremost Authority on Healing Herbs.* Emmaus, PA: Rodale Press, Inc., 1997.

"Immune-Boosting Recipes," adapted from *Creative Everyday Cooking.* Time-Life Books, 1990.

"Medicine in the New Millennium." *The Daytona Beach News Journal*, January 22, 2000.

Mowery, Daniel, Ph.D. *The Scientific Validation of Herbal Medicine*. Cormorant Books, 1986.

Page, Linda Rector, N.D., Ph.D. *Healthy Healing*, ninth edition. Healthy Healing Publications.

"Say Amen for Your Health's Sake." *Health Magazine*, October 1997.

Shamsuddin, A. M. et. al. "IP6: A Novel Anticancer Agent." *Life Sciences*, 61:343–54, 1997.

Walker, N. W., D.Sc. *Fresh Vegetable and Fruit Juices: What's Missing in Your Body?* Prescott, AZ: Norwalk Press, 1970.

APPENDIX B

PRODUCT SOURCES

THE FIRST 30 DAYS

Bragg's Liquid Aminos: Live Food Products, Santa Barbara, CA 93102. (800) 446-1990.

Carlson ACES and Carlson Multivitamin and Mineral Gelcaps: Carlson Laboratories, Inc., Arlington Heights, Illinois.

Kyo-Green: Wakunaga of America, 23501 Madero, Mission Viejo, CA 92691-2764. (800) 421-2998.

Nature's Secret Ultimate Cleanse: Nature's Secret, 5485 Conestoga Court, Boulder, CO 80301. (800) 525-9696; (303) 546-6306.

Stevia Extract Powder or Liquid: NOW Foods, 550 Mitchell Road, Glendale Heights, IL 60139. (800) 999-8069.

The products listed below can be found at almost any health food store across the nation:

- Roasted dandelion tea
- Soy cheese
- Rice milk
- Brown rice
- Maitake mushroom
- B-complex vitamin with pantothenic acid
- Green tea
- Rice cheese
- Soy milk
- Almond butter
- Sea salt (3 pounds)

THE NEXT 60 DAYS

Biotic silver: Candida Wellness Center, 4365 N. Bedford Dr., Provo, UT 84604. (800) 869-1613. Web site: www.candidayeast.com

Candistroy, Nature's Secret, Nature's Secret Ultimate Oil: Nature's Secret, 5485 Conestoga Court, Boulder, CO 80301. (800) 525-9696; (303) 546.6306.

Dr. Janet's Balanced by Nature Products: WTGL-TV52, Orlando, FL 32815. (407) 423-5200. Also available from Living Waters Health Foods, 141 W. Granada Blvd., Ormond Beach, FL 32174. (904) 672-6004.

Kyolic EPA: Wakunaga of America, 23501 Madero, Mission Viejo, CA 92691-2764. (800) 421-2998.

Lypo, Digest, Purify and Gastro Plant Enzymes: Enzymedica (Tom Bohager, director), 1970 Kings Hwy., Punta Gorda, FL 33980. (888) 918-1118.

90 DAYS

All products listed on the 90-Day Immune Maintenance and Body Balance protocol can be purchased at almost any health food store across the country, with the exception of CalMax, which can be purchased in bulk by calling (888) 677-9695. Single orders can be purchased from Living Waters Health Foods, 141 Granada Blvd., Ormond Beach, FL 32174; (904) 672-6004.

Dr. Janet's Balanced by Nature Products: WTGL-TV52, Orlando, FL 32805. (407) 423-5200. Also available from Living Waters Health Foods, 141 W. Granada Blvd., Ormond Beach, FL 32805. (904) 672-6004.

Lecithin: Lewis Laboratories International, Ltd., 49 Richmondville Ave., Westport, CT 06880.

NOTES

PART ONE: THE FIRST 30 DAYS

DETOXIFICATION

Quote from Leon Chaitow, N.D., D.O., London, England, is from *Alternative Medicine: The Definitive Guide,* compiled by the Burton Goldberg Group (Puyallup, WA: Future Medicine Publishing, Inc., 1993), 157.

IMMUNE RESPONSE

The Health Challenges Chart is adapted from a chart developed by Dean Black, Ph.D., author of *Health at the Crossroads.*

WATER

The Water Wisdom Chart is from *Rx for Cooking and Dietary Wellness,* James Balch, M.D. and Phyllis Balch, (n.p.: PAB Books, Inc., 1992).

Linda Rector Page, N.D., Ph.D., *Healthy Healing,* ninth edition (n.p.: Healthy Healing Publications).

SMOKING

The fourteen-day plan to stop smoking is adapted from *Dr. Berger's Immune Power Diet,* Stuart M. Berger, M.D. (New York: New American Library, 1985).

GREEN SUPERFOODS

James Balch, M.D. and Phyllis Balch, *Rx for Cooking and Dietary Wellness* (n.p., PAB Books, Inc., 1992).

POWER MUSHROOMS

Energy Times, November/December 1999.

Paul Stamets, *Growing Gourmet and Medicinal Mushrooms* (n.p.: Ten Speed Publishing, 1994).

The Townsend Letter, June 1998.

SCIENCE DOES AGREE: HAVE A CUP OF TEA

M. Serafini, "Red Wine, Tea and Antioxidants," *The Lancet,* 1994; 344:626.

C. S. Yang and Z. Y. Wang, "Tea and Cancer," *J. National Cancer Institute,* 85(13), 1038–1049.

THE EATING PLAN

The 90-Day Immune System Makeover eating plan has been adapted from *Healthy Healing,* ninth edition, Linda Rector Page, N.D., Ph.D., (n.p.: Healthy Healing Publications).

CHOOSE THE EXERCISE THAT BEST SUITS YOUR CURRENT HEALTH STATUS

Leslie Kaufman, "Your Prescription Is Ready," *Health Magazine,* October 1997.

SUMMARY—YOUR IMMUNITY: WHAT CAN GO WRONG?

American Journal of Clinical Nutrition, 1977: 613.

Lancet, 1977, 834–836.

American Journal of Clinical Nutrition, 50:851–867.

PART TWO: THE NEXT 60 DAYS

CALCIUM AND MAGNESIUM
Health Update: Featuring CalMax, with Dr. Janet Maccaro and Dr. Michael Pinkus,, produced by MEDIA Power, Portland, Maine, 1999.

CANDIDA AND CANDIDIASIS
W. G. Cook, M.D., "Candida Questionnaire and Score Sheet," *The Yeast Connection,* first edition (Jackson, TN: Professional Books, 1993), 29–33.

C. Orian Truss, M.D., *The Missing Diagnosis* (Birmingham, AL: 1983, 1986), 19–21.

ENZYMES—IMPROVED IMMUNE FUNCTION
M. Mamadou, M.D., "The White Paper," *Oral Enzymes: Facts and Concepts* (Houston, TX: Transformation Enzyme Corp.).

DicQie Fuller, Ph.D., D.Sc., *The Healing Power of Enzymes* (New York: Forbes Custom Publishing, 1998).

James Balch, M.D. and Phyllis Balch, *Prescription for Nutritional Healing* (New York: Avery Publishing Group, 1997).

THYROID HEALTH AND THE IMMUNE SYSTEM
Broda O. Barnes, M.D. and Lawrence Galton, *Hypothroidism: The Unsuspected Illness* (New York: Cromwell, 1976).

HORMONES AND HEALTH
John R. Lee., M.D., *What Your Doctor May Not Tell You About Menopause* (n.p.: Warner Books, 1996).

CATCH STRESS BEFORE IT CATCHES YOU
Hans Selye, *Stress Without Distress* (New York: New American Library, 1975)

James E. Marti, *Alternative Health Medicine Encyclopedia* (Detroit, MI: Visible Ink Press, 1995).

FOUR INDICATORS OF STRESS

Francisco Contreras, M.D., *Health in the 21st Century: Will Doctors Survive?* (Chula Vista, CA: Interpacific Press, 1997).

Quote from John Hibbs, N.D., is from *Alternative Medicine: The Definitive Guide,* compiled by the Burton Goldberg Group (Puyallup, WA: Future Medicine Publishing, Inc., 1993), 854.

STRESS: THE NATURAL APPROACH

Daniel O. Gagnon, *Healing Herbs for Your Nervous System* (Santa Fe, NM: Santa Fe Botanical Research and Educational Project, 1992).

WHAT DOES THE BIBLE SAY ABOUT STRESS, FEAR AND ANXIETY?

John Jeyseelan, president and CEO, Bethel Ministries, Inc., Daytona Beach, Florida.

STRESSED OUT: GRAB SOME GABA

Billie Jay Sahley, Ph.D., *Anxiety Epidemic* (San Antonio, TX: Pain and Stress Publications, 1997).

PART THREE: NINETY DAYS

IMMUNE-BOOSTING RECIPES

Adapted from *Creative Everyday Cooking* (Time-Life Books, 1990).

MEDICINE IN THE NEW MILLENNIUM

"Medicine in the New Millennium," *The Daytona Beach Journal,* January 22, 2000.

NEWS FLASH!
"Antibiotic-Resistant Bacteria Spreads," *Energy Times Magazine*, November/December 1989.

THE NEW CANCER FIGHTER—IP6
Abulkalam Shamsuddin et. al., "IP6: A Novel Anticancer Agent," *Life Sciences,* 61:343–54, 1997.

Abulkalam Shamsuddin, *IP6–Nature's Revolutionary Cancer Fighter* (n.p.: Kensington, 1998).

CAYENNE
Daniel Mowery, Ph.D., *The Scientific Validation of Herbal Medicine* (n.p.: Cormorant Books, 1986).

Your Walk With God Can Be Even Deeper...

With *Charisma* magazine, you'll be informed and inspired by the features and stories about what the Holy Spirit is doing in the lives of believers today.

Each issue:

- Brings you exclusive world-wide reports to rejoice over.
- Keeps you informed on the latest news from a Christian perspective.
- Includes miracle-filled testimonies to build your faith.
- Gives you access to relevant teaching and exhortation from the most respected Christian leaders of our day.

Call 1-800-829-3346 for 3 FREE trial issues

Offer #AOACHB

If you like what you see, then pay the invoice of $22.97 (**saving over 51% off the cover price**) and receive 9 more issues (12 in all). Otherwise, write "cancel" on the invoice, return it, and owe nothing.

Experience the Power of Spirit-Led Living

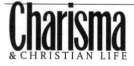

Charisma Offer #AOACHB
P.O. Box 420234
Palm Coast, Florida 32142-0234
www.charismamag.com

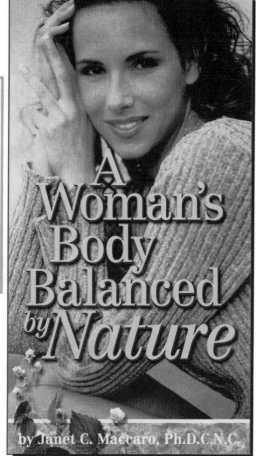

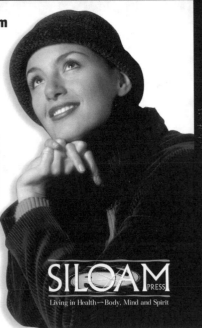